DR. COLBERT'S
HEALTH
ZONE
ESSENTIALS

DON COLBERT, MD

SILOAM

Dr. Colbert's Health Zone Essentials by Don Colbert, MD
Published by Siloam, an imprint of Charisma Media
1150 Greenwood Blvd., Lake Mary, Florida 32746

Unless otherwise noted, all Scripture quotations are taken from the New King James Version®. Copyright © 1982 by Thomas Nelson. Used by permission. All rights reserved.

Scripture quotations marked NLT are taken from the *Holy Bible*, New Living Translation, copyright ©1996, 2004, 2015 by Tyndale House Foundation. Used by permission of Tyndale House Publishers, Carol Stream, Illinois 60188. All rights reserved.

While the author has made every effort to provide accurate, up-to-date source information at the time of publication, statistics and other data are constantly updated. Neither the publisher nor the author assumes any responsibility for errors or for changes that occur after publication. Further, the publisher and author do not have any control over and do not assume any responsibility for third-party websites or their content.

For more resources like this, visit charismahouse.com, drcolbertbooks.com, and the author's website at drcolbert.com.

Cataloging-in-Publication Data is on file with the Library of Congress.
International Standard Book Number: 978-1-63641-351-8
E-book ISBN: 978-1-63641-352-5

1 2023
Printed in the United States of America

Most Charisma Media products are available at special quantity discounts for bulk purchase for sales promotions, premiums, fund-raising, and educational needs. For details, call us at (407) 333-0600 or visit our website at www.charismamedia.com.

This book contains the opinions and ideas of its author. It is solely for informational and educational purposes and should not be regarded as a substitute for professional medical treatment. The nature of your body's health condition is complex and unique. Therefore, you should consult

Portions of this book were previously published by Siloam as *Dr. Colbert's Healthy Brain Zone*, ISBN: 978-1-63641-109-5, copyright © 2023; *Beyond Keto*, ISBN: 978-1-63641-070-8, copyright © 2022; *Dr. Colbert's Healthy Gut Zone*, ISBN: 978-1-62999-981-4, copyright © 2021; *Dr. Colbert's Fasting Zone*, ISBN: 978-1-62999-764-2, copyright © 2020; and *Dr. Colbert's Hormone Health Zone*, ISBN: 978-1-62999-5731, copyright © 2019.

Some text of this book was rewritten by ChatGPT (and edited for content), OpenAI, August 22, 2023, https://chat.openai.com/chat.

CONTENTS

PART IV: SAFEGUARD YOUR BRAIN

INTRODUCTION

LIVE IN THE HEALTH ZONE!

I F YOU'VE EVER felt overwhelmed by the flood of health advice, unsure of where to turn amid the countless theories and trends, rest assured that you're not alone. The world of health is vast and complex, but I'm here to simplify it for you, to lead you into the *health zone essentials* of well-being where clarity, balance, and vibrancy thrive.

Over the years, I've dedicated my medical practice to offering not just solutions but a road map to true health. Through my books, I've sought to empower you with knowledge and wisdom, to help you take charge of your well-being in a world brimming with noise. *Dr. Colbert's Health Zone Essentials* is the culmination of decades of research, patient care, and personal commitment to holistic healing. It's a comprehensive guide that will illuminate your path to well-being, one step at a time.

Let me assure you, health isn't a collection of isolated fragments. It's a symphony of interconnected systems working together in harmony. That's why this book is built upon four key steps, each addressing a vital aspect of your well-being and elevating it to a new level. I wrote about these steps as individual books we call the Zone series, but I have always intended for them to work closely together. When followed in proper order, each Zone step builds upon the last, and together they create a pathway to optimum health. As a foundation of health, I recommend that you also read my book *The Seven Pillars of Health.*

Imagine this book as a treasure map, guiding your steps toward a destination called the Health Zone, where your energy soars, your mind is sharp, and your body thrives. It all begins with an exploration of the intricate world within you: your gut.

Step 1: Restore Your Gut for Optimal Wellness

Your gut is more than just a digestion center. It's a hub of vitality, influencing everything from your immunity to your mood. In the first part of this book, we'll delve into the profound significance of gut health. We'll explore the symbiotic relationship between your gut and your overall well-being. I'll guide you through the transformative power of nurturing your gut with healing food and supplements, and along the way you'll learn the five power tools for resetting your gut ecosystem, which is the foundation of the rest of your health.

Step 2: Embrace a Mediterranean-Keto Lifestyle

Once your gut is balanced and restored, you must eat a healthy diet to keep it that way. Step 2 is a feast of insights that marry the fat-burning power of the keto diet with the wisdom of the Mediterranean lifestyle. This fusion creates a symphony of flavors that nourish not only your body but also your brain. I've led many patients through the keto plan and have learned the best ways to make it even healthier and more effective by blending it with key principles from the timeless truth of the Mediterranean diet. You'll also discover the power of intermittent fasting to unlock your body's potential for energy, balance, and longevity.

Step 3: Make a Great Life With Hormone Optimization

As we reach new heights of well-being, we'll encounter the symphony of hormones that orchestrate your bodily functions. Step 3 illuminates the importance of hormonal balance in achieving vibrant health. We'll journey through natural approaches to hormone optimization for both men and women, delving into hormone replacement protocols and the vital role of understanding your body's unique needs. Whether you're navigating hormonal shifts or seeking vitality, this part will guide you toward optimal hormone health.

STEP 4: SAFEGUARD YOUR BRAIN

The pinnacle of our journey brings us to the brain—the epicenter of your existence. In step 4 we'll explore the intricate landscape of brain protection. Cognitive vitality is essential for a life well lived, and I'll unveil how you can preserve and enhance your brain's health through nutritional choices, holistic practices, and a commitment to mental wellness.

Appendix A provides you with nutritional guidelines and my favorite Mediterranean-keto recipes. This practical resource is your culinary companion, offering a collection of nourishing recipes that align with the approach I wrote about in my book *Beyond Keto*. These recipes encompass the best of both dietary paradigms, ensuring that your path to the Health Zone is a delicious and satisfying one.

Appendix B offers you further resources for the *Health Zone Essentials* lifestyle. You'll find my recommendations for the right tests and blood work to ask for as you start your journey, the best supplements for restoring balance and optimizing your health, and the best way to access doctors and other resources that will help you on your Health Zone journey.

CRAFTING YOUR PERSONALIZED HEALTH ZONE

Now that you have a glimpse of the four steps that compose this book, I encourage you to envision yourself taking these steps on the path to well-being. Picture yourself in each step—healing your gut; embracing a Mediterranean-keto diet and elevating your healthy lifestyle through fasting, exercise, and other important health habits; balancing your hormones; and nurturing your brain. Imagine the vitality that will flow through you, the energy that will ignite your days, and the clarity that will guide your decisions.

As you turn each page, remember that you're not alone on this journey. I'm here, your guide and companion, sharing the knowledge that has transformed the lives of countless individuals. But remember, this isn't a passive experience—it's an empowering one. I invite you to take notes, highlight insights, and engage with the practices presented. Craft your own wellness plan, incorporating the wisdom of each part.

By the time you reach the end of this book, you'll have a comprehensive plan tailored to your unique needs. You'll possess the tools to heal, nourish, and elevate your body, mind, and spirit. Your journey through the Health Zone essentials will be nothing short of transformative, and I'm honored to be with you every step of the way.

So let's embark on this journey together, live in the Health Zone, and embrace a life of total wellness.

PART I
RESTORE YOUR GUT FOR OPTIMAL WELLNESS

CHAPTER 1

THE FOUNDATION OF HEALTH: YOUR GUT

WELCOME TO THE cornerstone of your journey to better health—the world of gut health. While it might not be the most glamorous topic, your gut is a critically important part of your overall health, affecting everything from your immune system to your mood.

Your gut is a definite hero for your health, working diligently behind the scenes to bolster your overall well-being. In this chapter we will look at the critical importance of having a healthy gut and its impact on multiple dimensions of your health.

THE UNSUNG HERO OF HEALTH

In all the talk about staying healthy, people don't usually pay much attention to the gut. But the importance of your gut can't be overstated. It's like a hidden world that's full of connections that affect your overall health, not just digestion, in many ways. Your gut emerges as the unsung hero of your holistic health, orchestrating an intricate network known as the gut-body axis. This axis is the conduit through which your gut communicates with various organs and systems, including your immune system and your hormones; it even influences your emotions and how your body uses energy.

Simply put, your gut health has a significant impact on how good you feel overall. It makes everything work well and causes you to feel alive and well.

A VITAL CONNECTION

Imagine your gut as the leader of a large orchestra, directing a beautiful show of activities that do more than just digest food. Scientists call this the gut-body axis. It's like the different instruments in an orchestra working together to make great music. In the same way the different instruments in an orchestra work together to make great music, this axis is like a network of pathways that connect your gut to many different parts of your body. Your gut is like the conductor of this orchestra, making sure everything works well. It controls a variety of important functions that affect how you feel and how healthy you are.

Think of your digestive system as a complex system of roads connecting your gut to different parts of your body. Just as phones and computers send messages through networks, your gut communicates with other important parts of your body through these pathways. This communication affects how your immune system functions, how your hormones work, how your body uses energy, and even how you feel emotionally. All these systems are connected and depend on your gut being healthy. This is why taking care of your gut is so important.

This section talks about how your gut connects to different parts of your body and how taking care of it is key to being healthy. As you learn more, you'll find out ways to keep this network strong, which will help you stay well and happy.

MICROSCOPIC HEROES

If you were to explore the inside of your gut, you'd find it full of tiny living things called microorganisms. These little guys, known as your gut microbiota, might seem small, but they're really important for your health. They live in your digestive system and do much more than just help you digest food. To truly comprehend the importance of these microorganisms, it's essential to recognize their pivotal role in maintaining the delicate balance and vitality of your gut environment.

Among the inhabitants of your gut microbiota, beneficial bacteria emerge as the unsung heroes of your gut's symphony. While their significance might not be immediately apparent, these tiny allies play an indispensable role in multiple aspects of your health. They are the diligent workers that aid in digestion, breaking down complex food particles and making vital nutrients more accessible to your body. But their contributions don't stop there—these beneficial bacteria also produce an array of compounds that have far-reaching effects. From regulating inflammation to fostering a gut environment that supports immune function, these microorganisms operate as silent champions, working tirelessly to maintain balance within your body.

Just as a symphony relies on each instrument playing its part, your gut ecosystem thrives on balance. An imbalance in your gut microbiota can lead to a variety of health issues, disrupting the equilibrium that ensures your well-being. When harmful microorganisms gain the upper hand, they can lead to a range of complications, from digestive discomfort to compromised immune function. Imbalances have been associated with conditions such as irritable bowel syndrome (IBS), inflammatory bowel disease (IBD), and even mental health disorders.

Knowing how important these tiny living beneficial microbes are and how they need to work together helps you understand why you should take care of them.

Your Second Brain

The gastrointestinal (GI) system is sometimes referred to as the "second brain" due to its complex and intricate neural network, also known as the enteric nervous system. This extensive network of neurons is found within the walls of the gastrointestinal tract and is capable of independently controlling various digestive processes. The enteric nervous system communicates with the central nervous system (the brain and spinal cord) through a bidirectional pathway known as the gut-brain axis.

The gut-brain axis is a fascinating and intricate connection that highlights the two-way communication between the gut and the brain. Notably, the gut can send signals to the brain that influence mood, emotions, and even cognitive functions. This connection has led to the observation that the gut is like a "second brain" because of its ability to affect how you feel and think.

Research into the gut-brain axis continues to uncover the extent of this connection and its implications for both physical and mental health. Factors such as the gut microbiota, neurotransmitter production, and immune responses within the gut play a role in this complex relationship. This connection again underscores the importance of the gut.

THE HEALTHY GUT ZONE APPROACH

In my book *Dr. Colbert's Healthy Gut Zone*, I discuss in more detail the causes of imbalances in the gut and the illnesses an unhealthy gut can cause. I encourage you to read it if you want a fuller understanding of your digestive health. As we move forward in this book, we'll be expediting the path to health by diving into the healthy gut protocols. We'll be creating a plan to restore your gut and get it functioning at its prime. And you'll discover how your dietary choices and lifestyle practices contribute to the health of this complex system.

Taking care of your gut ecosystem starts with making smart choices about what you eat. These choices do more than just improve satiety; they actually help your gut work smoothly. An important part of this journey is adding certain foods to your diet that are full of prebiotics and probiotics. Prebiotics—found in things such as garlic, onions, and artichokes—support the helpful bacteria in your gut. Alongside this, you have probiotics, which are in foods such as yogurt, kefir, and fermented veggies. These foods introduce live beneficial bacteria to your gut, enriching its microbial diversity.

However, having a healthy gut doesn't rely solely on what you consume. There are other habits that play a pivotal role. Think of these habits as protectors of the intricate ecosystem inside you. Staying hydrated, getting regular exercise, managing stress, and getting enough sleep all help your gut-body axis stay strong. Each habit complements the others, creating a well-rounded approach that strengthens your gut ecosystem, thereby enhancing its capacity to support your overall well-being. From fermented foods to dietary fiber, you have a range of options that can help your gut thrive and make your whole body feel full of life.

THE RIPPLE EFFECT: TOTAL WELLNESS FROM WITHIN

When you begin your journey toward improving your gut health, you set off a chain reaction of positive changes that go way beyond just your digestion. Think of it like dropping a pebble into a calm pond. Each little ripple shows something changing inside your body. When you take good care of your gut, you're actually starting a chain of improvements that spread to every part of your body.

By giving your gut some attention, you're unlocking numerous benefits that all add up to making you feel better. Your ability to digest foods improves, which means smoother digestion and your body can use important nutrients better. It's not just about what you eat; it's about making sure your body can really digest and absorb the nutrients from the food you consume. Plus, when you make choices to improve your gut health, your immune system—the system that keeps you healthy—gets stronger, bolstering its ability to protect you from external threats.

Always remember, a healthy gut is where a vibrant life starts. From helping your immune system work better to stabilizing your mood to sharpening your mind and improving your digestion, taking care of your gut sparks a real transformation.

CHAPTER 2

MAKE YOUR PLAN

DEALING WITH ANY illness or affliction is a daunting experience. When I grappled with psoriasis, it nearly pushed me to my limits. I fought against it every single day for years. And on top of the physical discomfort, the condition made me feel embarrassed, like I couldn't help my patients because I couldn't even help myself. But surprisingly, I found a solution for my psoriasis that was much simpler, cheaper, and less disruptive than I ever anticipated. Once I fixed the issues in my gut, my psoriasis gradually faded away, revealing just how much gut health can affect our well-being.

Chances are you're reading this book because you or someone dear to you is wrestling with some type of health condition you're hoping will improve. I have seen many lives radically changed for the better by applying the principles of my *Healthy Gut Zone* book. It's impossible to guarantee anything in the medical profession, of course. But I can say that I'm no longer surprised to hear folks sharing stories of big improvements or even complete turnarounds of conditions, diagnoses, or situations once deemed irreversible. These success stories usually begin when people restore their gut health.

When your gut heals, you usually get incredible health benefits. As the foundation to so much, whether good or bad, the gut plays a surprisingly pivotal role in basically every disease known to man. In short, a healthy gut can usher in health and healing literally from head to toe. So no matter why you picked up this book, let's get your gut healthy again. Then you can see what happens after that!

Start by Stopping

It might sound counterintuitive, but embarking on the path to gut health starts with hitting the brakes. It's time to halt those eating, drinking, or other habits that might be unsettling your GI tract. By eliminating the culprits behind inflammation and leaky gut, you're giving your body a chance to break free of its ongoing cycle. Keep in mind, our bodies often crave the very foods that invite inflammation and disease.

In the following chart is my list of things you should try to avoid.

WHAT TO AVOID

» *alcohol (best to remove entirely)*

» *antibiotics*

» *anti-inflammatory medications (such as aspirin, Advil, Motrin, Aleve, etc.)*

» *artificial sweeteners*

» *chlorinated water*

» *dairy (cheese, milk, cream, butter, yogurt, etc.)*

» *excessive meats, especially processed meats and fatty meats*

» *gluten (bread, pasta, bagels, rolls, biscuits, etc.)*

» *GMO food*

» *high-lectin food (usually can add some back in two to three months—more on this later). Those under eighteen should consume adequate healthy starches and carbohydrates.*

» *medications for GERD and acid-blocking meds*

» *processed food (most food in a box) and excessive starches and carbs (potatoes, rice, corn). Limit starches to the size of a tennis ball or less and only one per meal (if over eighteen).*

> » *saturated fats (reduce or eliminate), especially butter, cheese, cream, and coconut oil*
>
> » *sugar*
>
> » *Additionally, I always recommend thoroughly rinsing the mouth after using fluoride toothpaste since fluoride kills good bacteria if swallowed. Making the switch from fluoride toothpaste to a natural option might be beneficial for some.*

From a technical standpoint, virtually everything listed here tends to harm the gut, fuel gut inflammation, or promote undesirable bacteria dwelling in your gut. Clearly, that's not what you're aiming for.

While this list might not be a guaranteed cure-all, it often has an immediate or nearly immediate impact on the symptoms many patients face. Prioritizing the nourishment of beneficial bacteria is your goal, as these are the allies striving to promote your overall well-being. Kicking out the substances that fuel undesirable bacteria is an excellent first step. That's why I recommend that you start by stopping.

ADD THE RIGHT NUTRIENTS TO YOUR GUT

Getting your gut health back on track doesn't depend on using a lot of fancy supplements. The real key to fixing your gut is to stop using medicines and eating foods that harm it. You don't have to spend a ton of money on rare supplements—that's not the path we're taking here.

Healing your gut is mainly about giving it the essential nutrients it needs. While some supplements can help, most of what your gut needs will come from eating foods that have what it craves.

The goal is to restore a proper balance of beneficial bacteria, eradicate harmful microbes, facilitate the healing of your gut lining, and alleviate inflammation. To accomplish this, your dietary focus will typically need to include these elements: fiber, polyphenols, prebiotics, and probiotics. I'll discuss these in detail later.

Depending on your specific symptoms, health issues, or conditions, supplements can provide added and targeted benefits. In such cases, the following supplements might offer valuable support:

- colostrum (to repair leaky gut), if not sensitive to dairy
- deglycyrrhizinated licorice (DGL, to repair leaky gut)
- herbs (slippery elm, marshmallow root, and aloe vera to soothe and protect the gut and boost mucus production)
- hydrolyzed collagen (to help repair leaky gut)
- L-glutamine (to help repair leaky gut)
- magnesium (to improve bowel motility)
- omega-3 (to help quench inflammation and repair the gut)
- vitamin D_3 (to help regulate gut bacteria)
- zinc (to improve the barrier function of the gut)

Incorporating fermented food and resistant starches into your diet, if you haven't already, is crucial. These choices provide remarkable benefits to the good bacteria in your gut. The good news is that when you nourish your gut with the right food and eliminate problematic elements, your gut often can self-heal. The process is surprisingly straightforward.

You might find that some of the food and drinks you desire are off the table (no pun intended), or you might need to cut back considerably. Yet your overall well-being hinges on revitalizing your gut, so the effort is certainly worth it!

What could be unsettling your colon and leading to constipation? Among the common culprits I often come across are excessive stress, a sluggish or underactive thyroid, and a deficiency in essentials such as exercise, fiber, fluids, and magnesium.

Most people fall short of drinking enough water (a minimum of eight cups daily, although greater fluid intake is recommended[1]). However, maintaining adequate hydration is quite achievable.

When it comes to fiber and magnesium, we typically don't get ample amounts through our diet. This essentially leaves the supplementation route as our only option. American adults eat 15–16 grams of fiber a day on average.[2] For adults under the age of fifty, the Institute of Medicine suggests a daily fiber intake of 26 grams for women and 38 grams for men. For those over age fifty, it is 21 grams for women and 30 grams for men.[3]

I have found that most of my patients don't get enough fiber and magnesium. Chances are you might be facing similar deficiencies. Shockingly, around 50 percent of the US population is deficient in magnesium.[4] Boosting your magnesium levels is achievable by eating food such as spinach, kale, almonds, dark chocolate, and avocados—these choices are also kind to your gut. In a mere ounce of almonds, you'll find 80 milligrams of magnesium. Conversely, food rich in magnesium but less friendly to your gut includes options such as whole wheat, black beans, and edamame. For adults, the advised daily magnesium intake ranges from 310 to 420 milligrams, depending on age and gender.[5]

Incorporate some probiotics and prebiotics, and you're taking significant steps toward healing your gut.

GET USED TO EATING HEALTHY FOOD

Adopting a gut-friendly diet isn't as challenging or unconventional as it might appear to some. Here's a rundown of natural food that would be beneficial in your diet:

- **Avocado:** This stands out as possibly the finest fruit ever cultivated. Unlike most fruits that contain sugar, which feeds bad gut bacteria, avocados are almost sugar-free. They pack in good fats (avocado oil is highly beneficial), fiber (a vital component often lacking in diets), magnesium, and potassium. Note, though, that avocados can trigger excess gas in individuals with IBS and small intestinal bacterial overgrowth (SIBO) due to their high fermentable oligo-saccharides, disaccharides, monosaccharides, and polyols (FODMAP) content. If you're considering them, start slowly.

- **Oils:** Opt for organic extra-virgin avocado and olive oils that come loaded with vitamins, minerals, and polyphenols— all nutrients your gut continually craves. Make liberal use of both these oils in your meals. Olive oil notably reduces inflammation,[6] and its polyphenols aid in gut healing.

- **Greens:** Embrace a variety of greens, especially since you'll be consuming numerous salads. Ranging from romaine lettuce to arugula, kohlrabi, and spinach, these veggies are lectin-free[7]—an optimal choice for your gut health. Drizzle them generously with avocado or olive oil.

- **Resistant starches:** Instead of the usual suspects, such as white or red potatoes, shift your focus to sweet potatoes, yucca, or taro root. However, limit portions to half a cup since they're rich in carbs. These alternatives align with what your gut craves: minimal sugar content and abundant fiber, vitamins, and minerals.

- **Lean, grass-fed meat and wild low-mercury fish:** While meat is an excellent protein source, excessive consumption can slow digestion. Prioritize gut-friendly meats such as wild fish (e.g., Alaskan salmon, sardines), organic range-fed poultry (e.g., chicken, turkey), and grass-fed and grass-finished beef. Aim for a balance of two-thirds veggies and one-fourth to one-third meat (two to three ounces for women, three to six ounces for men) during meals. Processed meats such as bacon and sausages should be avoided.

- **Starchy alternatives:** When it comes to staples such as bread, pasta, corn, and rice, opt for alternatives such as millet bread or those crafted from almond flour, coconut flour, or cassava flour. Similarly, consider cassava tortillas as an option. (See appendix A.)

Your gut prefers this kind of thinking: "Feed me food low in sugars and carbs, brimming with fiber, probiotics, prebiotics, and polyphenols, and I will be content. When I'm content, your health thrives. And with thriving health, you are happy."

This is the fundamental goal when it comes to choosing food, eating healthily, and nourishing your gut. The process should not be overly complicated or arduous; otherwise, it's unlikely to be followed. Thankfully, your gut is easy to please.

In this chapter we've covered the place to start (by stopping) and first steps forward. We will delve further into the Health Zone in the next chapter as I introduce you to five power tools for your gut. These strategies are designed to empower you on your journey toward a healthier, happier you. So let's move on to explore the five fundamental tools for cultivating a thriving gut ecosystem.

CHAPTER 3

FIVE POWER TOOLS TO NOURISH YOUR GUT

I'M GOING TO make a bold statement. Every day I see patients who are grappling with various symptoms, and I firmly believe that every one of them would likely see improvement if they took action to restore their gut health and adopted a diet rich in gut-friendly elements such as fiber, probiotics, prebiotics, and polyphenols. A majority of symptoms would probably go away, usually carrying with them any underlying sicknesses and diseases.

That's how powerful the gut is. Once it's revitalized, it can potentially harmonize the rest of your body! If your focus is on enhancing your gut health, the following pages outline five "gut power tools"—tried and true methods that are known to be profoundly beneficial for your gut.

GUT POWER TOOL 1: FIBER

The first gut power tool is none other than good old fiber—not the kind derived from beans, wheat bran, or grains laden with lectins, but rather psyllium husk powder. Although it might not seem exciting or cool, it takes center stage in the restoration of your gut health.

As I mentioned earlier, few people get enough fiber in their diets. Scarcely any of my patients consistently meet their fiber needs, and a mere 5 percent of Americans fulfill the requirements for adequate fiber intake.[1] Therefore, it's common to see patients with low-fiber symptoms such as constipation, inability to lose weight, low energy, hunger soon after eating, and craving between meals.[2]

Of course, you can't blame everything on fiber, as it's merely a single component within the intricate puzzle of a healthy gut. But consuming the right sources of fiber in the right amounts can potentially reset your gut health and may also help control blood sugar levels; lower blood pressure and cholesterol; make you feel full longer, causing you to reduce food intake and lose weight; normalize bowel movements; lower risk of heart disease; minimize hemorrhoids; and help prevent diverticular disease.[3]

I recommend 30–35 grams of fiber per day, but start low and go slow to avoid bloating and gas. Technically, fiber comes in two different forms: soluble and insoluble. Your body needs both.

Sources of these fibers are not typically gut friendly, so my top recommendation for soluble fiber intake is psyllium husk powder. Psyllium is mainly a soluble fiber with some insoluble fiber from the seed husks of the plant *Plantago ovata*.

Many laxative or fiber mixes claim to provide your body with the fiber it needs. Though that might be true, it is the other ingredients (especially sugars and artificial sweeteners) that concern me. You can buy the psyllium husk powder by itself, with nothing else added to it. It is inexpensive, but do not buy the psyllium husk powder with sugar, NutraSweet, or Splenda. (For those who dislike the taste, we have a great-tasting, healthy fiber listed in appendix B.)

Start with one-half teaspoon of psyllium husk powder in a four-ounce glass of cold filtered water after breakfast once a day, eventually working up to twice a day, after breakfast and after dinner. If you are new to taking fiber, start low and go slow, such as one-fourth teaspoon after breakfast. If no gas or bloating occurs, then slowly work your way up to a full or heaping teaspoon once or twice a day. (On a side note, you will want to rinse your glass carefully, or the fiber will stick.)

For insoluble fiber, I suggest nuts, nut butters, artichoke, cauliflower, broccoli, and other cruciferous veggies. The veggie stems have the most insoluble fiber, so be sure to eat those as well.

More to know about fiber

Constipation is terrible news for your gut. To stop being constipated, taking one teaspoon to one heaping teaspoon of psyllium husk powder after breakfast and/or dinner will usually do the trick if you are drinking enough water (at least eight cups per day). Eventually, aim for 25–35 grams a day, and you can't go wrong. Add that to sufficient water intake, and you will often begin to see the magic of fiber after a week or two.

We all need fiber, but if you suffer from IBS, small intestinal fungal overgrowth (SIFO), SIBO, or IBD, then fiber may cause bloating and gas. If you have colitis or Crohn's disease, fiber may cause a flare-up. What is the answer? Some doctors recommend avoiding fiber altogether until the patient's ailment, such as SIBO, is under control. It is up to you, but I tell my patients to start low and go slow. Your gut needs the many benefits of fiber, but if it takes you a while to get there, that is fine.

GUT POWER TOOL 2: PROBIOTICS

The second gut power tool is probiotics. Probiotics are live microorganisms, typically bacteria or yeast, that offer potential health benefits when consumed in adequate amounts. Found in certain food and supplements, these beneficial microorganisms aim to support the balance of gut bacteria and promote overall digestive and immune health.

You can take probiotics as supplements in liquid, pill, or powder form, but probiotics are also found in fermented food such as kefir, kimchi, kombucha, miso, natto, pickles, sauerkraut, tempeh, traditional buttermilk, and yogurt. Dairy is harmful and inflammatory to many of my patients' GI tracts. If lactose intolerance is a concern, or you are sensitive to dairy, opt for coconut kefir or coconut yogurt, or goat or sheep yogurt or kefir. Regardless of your preference, you have an abundance of options that are full of probiotics and extremely healthy for your gut.

COMMON PROBIOTICS

This is a list of gut-friendly probiotics that are readily available in food or supplements.

» *Lactobacillus acidophilus: helps decrease bad bacteria growth, helps maintain gut bacteria balance, helps reduce yeast infections*[4]

» *Lactobacillus brevis: helps reduce lipopolysaccharide (LPS), strengthens gut wall, improves immune function*[5]

» *Lactobacillus casei: helps heal infectious diarrhea*[6]

» *Lactobacillus gasseri: helps treat H. pylori*[7]

» *Lactobacillus plantarum: helps heal infectious diarrhea, helps decrease inflammation, helps maintain gut bacteria balance*[8]

» *Lactobacillus rhamnosus: helps prevent diarrhea*[9]

» *Lactobacillus salivarius: helps reduce gas*[10]

» *Streptococcus thermophilus: helps digest lactose*[11]

» *Bifidobacterium bifidum: is beneficial for the immune system*[12]

» *Bifidobacterium infantis: helps with IBS*[13]

» *Bifidobacterium longum: helps prevent diarrhea and constipation, helps improve lactose tolerance*[14]

» *Bifidobacterium lactis: helps decrease bloating, strengthens gut wall, helps boost immunity*[15]

» *Saccharomyces boulardii: helps heal infectious diarrhea*[16]

Thousands of species of bacteria live in the world and in your gut—many of them good and beneficial. Probiotics crowd out the bad bacteria in your gut and stop them from colonizing. This minimizes ongoing damage to your gut while increasing the number of good bacteria. The good bacteria then have room to grow and multiply, bringing healing to your gut and body.

But probiotics are something that you continually need to eat or take as supplements. One glass of goat milk kefir or one helping of sauerkraut is good for your gut, but just as with fiber, you need a daily intake of probiotics for your gut health. (See appendix B for powerful probiotics that I recommend to many of my patients.)

As you work to include probiotics in your diet daily, keep in mind that it is good to shake things up a bit. Rotating probiotics after three to six months is recommended to keep your gut's microbiome diverse and healthy.[17] The more you do this naturally with the food you eat, the happier your gut will be.

Probiotics help repair the gut lining, which immediately decreases inflammation. When the inflammation subsides, the symptoms usually disappear. This also typically helps reduce every related risk of disease. For most people, eating food with probiotics or taking probiotic supplements is more than sufficient. Probiotics may help boost one's immune system and protect one against infections. Statistics show that probiotics help train our immune system.

Further benefits of probiotics

Probiotics have also been found to help with acne, antibiotic-associated diarrhea (AAD), bacterial vaginosis (BV), dysbiosis, infectious diarrhea, IBD, IBS, leaky gut, sinus infections, traveler's diarrhea, urinary tract infections (UTIs), and yeast infections.[18]

But that's not all. Probiotics are used to fight depression.[19] Probiotics (called psychobiotics) are being used to improve and support mental health.[20] Probiotics (*Lactobacillus brevis* and *plantarum*, in particular) are used to increase brain-derived neurotrophic factor (BDNF), a brain-growth hormone.[21] Probiotics also are used to improve your immune system[22] and reduce LPS, an endotoxin that is bad for your gut and gut wall.[23]

If you are thinking, "What about probiotics and weight loss?" you are right on target. Dr. Steven Gundry clearly states, "The organisms in your intestines control how skinny or fat you will be."[24] The bacteria in your gut play a huge role in weight loss and weight gain.

GUT POWER TOOL 3: PREBIOTICS

The third gut power tool is prebiotics. Like probiotics, prebiotics are incredibly beneficial to your gut's microbiome and your entire GI tract. Prebiotics are a type of dietary fiber that serve as nourishment for beneficial gut bacteria. They are nondigestible compounds found in certain food, particularly plant-based sources such as fruits, vegetables, whole grains, and legumes. By providing a supportive environment for good bacteria to flourish, prebiotics indirectly promote gut health and overall well-being.

Though prebiotics are available in supplement form, the most common way to get prebiotics is through the food we eat—asparagus, green bananas, carrots, cocoa, coconut meat and milk, dandelion greens, flax-seeds, garlic, Jerusalem artichokes, leeks, onions, radishes, and seaweed are gut-friendly sources. Green bananas have an extra benefit that we will discuss in gut power tool 5.

Using prebiotics to help your gut

Achieving gut health involves supplying your gut with the necessary nutrients once bloating and gas have been managed. This entails incorporating prebiotics, as these compounds fuel beneficial bacteria, enabling them to proliferate and contribute to holistic well-being.

Within our gut reside two primary types of microbes—Firmicutes and Bacteroidetes. Although it's crucial to maintain Firmicutes for the health of the gastrointestinal tract, overpopulation beyond Bacteroidetes usually results in weight gain. Conversely, when Bacteroidetes dominate, weight loss and a leaner profile typically follow suit. A diet laden with sugar, carbs, and starches but low in fiber tends to favor Firmicutes growth, correlating with weight gain. Conversely, a Healthy Gut Zone diet, rich in fiber and prebiotics while low in sugar, carbs, and starches, promotes the dominance of Bacteroidetes and facilitates weight loss.

An added benefit of prebiotics is their role in generating butyrate, a short-chain fatty acid that holds significant benefits for your gut. Butyrate not only serves as fuel for colon cells but also exhibits anti-inflammatory properties. This reduction in inflammation can be transformative for many individuals, altering the course of their health. Butyrate also supports the immune system and safeguards against specific digestive tract ailments. The more butyrate in your gut, the better off you will be.

Moreover, prebiotics contribute to enhanced energy levels, weight loss, and better absorption of minerals such as magnesium and calcium; counteract common negative effects of stomach acid blockers; fortify existing gut probiotics; and suppress hunger.

When advising my patients, I recommend aiming for around 12 grams of prebiotics daily once the issues of gas and bloating have subsided. Wondering how to quantify that? If you're already incorporating the necessary fiber and probiotics into your diet, introducing roughly a handful of prebiotic-rich food should suffice. Feel free to include an abundance of naturally prebiotic-packed vegetables in your salads or cooked dishes— the more this practice becomes habitual, the better.

However, a word of caution for individuals diagnosed with SIBO, SIFO, or IBD (Crohn's or ulcerative colitis). Although prebiotics are inherently beneficial, they might trigger increased bloating and gas for some. In such cases, discontinuing prebiotic supplements is advisable. Gradually introducing natural prebiotic food might be a better approach, beginning with modest amounts and proceeding gradually. As your gut health improves through your restoration efforts, the likelihood is that over time, bloating and gas will diminish, allowing you to enjoy prebiotics without such discomfort.

GUT POWER TOOL 4: POLYPHENOLS

Polyphenols are a class of naturally occurring compounds found in various plant-based food. They are known for their potent antioxidant properties, which contribute to their potential health benefits. Polyphenols are abundant in fruits, vegetables, whole grains, nuts, seeds, tea, and certain beverages such as red wine and coffee. Consuming food rich in polyphenols has been linked to various health advantages, including reduced inflammation, improved heart health, and enhanced gut function.

POLYPHENOLS

Polyphenols are natural antioxidant compounds that protect us from toxins, prevent blood clots, promote gut health, reduce cell damage, and more. There are two main classes:

1. *Flavonoids (60 percent of polyphenols)*

2. *Phenolic acids (30 percent of polyphenols)*

You can eat the following healthy polyphenols as much as you like: berries (blueberries, raspberries, blackberries, ¼–½ cup a day), black tea, coffee, dark chocolate (72 percent cacao or more), green tea, and olive oils and olives (especially high-phenolic olive oil and oleocanthal). One of the most common polyphenols from this list is chlorogenic acid, from coffee. There are also quite a few polyphenol supplements to choose from, such as grapeseed extract, green tea extract, and pine bark extract.

As with our other gut power tools, not every source of polyphenols is recommendable if you are working to restore your gut health. Staying low sugar/low fructose means avoiding all or most fruits and all fruit juices. Avoid grains and beans (because of lectins), but most nuts, spices, and seasonings are fine.

For me, extra-virgin olive oil is the primary source of polyphenols, as it makes the perfect salad dressing and can be drizzled over most cooked food and added to soup.

Olive oil's best-kept secret: oleocanthal

One of the many phenolic compounds is oleocanthal, one of the most powerful phytonutrients in the world. Because oleocanthal is so good for you, it has been highly investigated and researched. It was discovered in 1993, defined in 2005, and found (among many other things) to be like liquid ibuprofen.[25] This oleocanthal is more active than many medications, and it is an anti-inflammatory and a pain reliever. It's also 100 percent natural, which means you get the ibuprofen benefit without any of the side effects.

Interestingly, the only known source for this special oleocanthal polyphenol is extra-virgin olive oil. It is found nowhere else. Oleocanthal is found in the highest concentrations in extra-virgin olive oil from certain locations in Greece.

GUT POWER TOOL 5: RESISTANT STARCHES

The fifth and final gut power tool is resistant starches. Resistant starches are a type of dietary carbohydrate that resists digestion in the small intestine and reaches the large intestine mostly unchanged. This unique characteristic allows them to serve as a source of nourishment for beneficial gut bacteria, promoting their growth and activity. Resistant starches are found in food such as undercooked potatoes, green bananas, legumes, and some whole grains. They offer several potential health benefits, including improved gut health, enhanced insulin sensitivity, and better blood sugar control.

Not every carb is a resistant starch. In fact, decreasing your carb intake to lower sugars is a necessary part of giving your gut time to heal. The bad bacteria thrive in a sugar-rich environment, while the good bacteria need a low-sugar environment to thrive.

So where do you find these resistant starches? Familiar food sources include sweet potatoes, yams, green (not fully ripened) bananas, green mangos, green papaya, and green plantains. You are no doubt thinking (as with the lists of options for fiber, probiotics, prebiotics, and polyphenols) that not every option for resistant starches is going to be the right choice while you are trying to restore your gut health. That is true.

For the first month or two you should avoid beans, peas, and lentils while you are focusing on restoring your gut, and then follow the instructions for soaking and properly cooking them. Corn, oats, barley, and rice have a lot of carbs and lectins. I would avoid them for now as well.

As for the fruits, when the fruit is fully ripened, both the sugar/fructose content and lectin content are high. Eating the green fruit bypasses the sugar/fructose and lectins and provides you with a great source of resistant starches. These fruits are good for your gut, but only when they are green. Sliced in bite-size pieces, they are a great topping on salads. That is always my recommendation for getting these resistant starches into a daily diet routine.

Flours from green bananas and plantains are also available. They are great for cooking or baking, and the resistant starches feed the good bacteria in your gut.

CHAPTER 4

RESTORE GUT HEALTH WITH FOOD

EVERY PATIENT OF mine who has taken the initiative to enhance their gut health has reaped multiple health benefits directly linked to their efforts. As I've endeavored to convey throughout this book, healing your gut translates to a victory for your entire body. The foundation of a healthy body is a healthy gut.

I am not promising that the Healthy Gut Zone diet will eradicate every disease, malady, discomfort, or symptom. Nevertheless, my experiences with patients have yielded many positive outcomes, instances where favorable prognoses emerged despite prior discouraging initial diagnoses. It's this track record that urges me to advocate giving it a try. Eating according to my recommendations in this chapter is aimed at three goals, which we will do simultaneously: feed the good bacteria, starve the bad bacteria, and give your gut a rest so it can restore itself.

FEEDING THE GOOD

To feed the good bacteria in your gut what they need to be healthy and effective, you will want to eat gut-friendly food. Veggies are the base of the Healthy Gut Zone diet. You want about one-half to two-thirds of each lunch and dinner to be raw or cooked veggies because that is what your gut needs the most. Protein from a variety of sources is a side but vitally important. Everything else (low-sugar fruits, healthy fats, resistant starches) is a complementary but necessary addition. All combined, your gut bacteria thrive on this mix of ingredients. Here's a list of food to eat as you focus on feeding the good bacteria to restore your gut health.

GUT-HEALING FOOD

Put these food options at the top of your shopping list while on the Healthy Gut Zone diet.

Veggies: *artichokes, arugula, asparagus, basil, beets, bok choy, broccoli, brussels sprouts, cabbage (Chinese, green, red), carrots, cauliflower, celery, chives, cilantro, cucumbers (if peeled and deseeded), garlic, greens (collard, dandelion, field, mustard), kale, kimchi, kohlrabi, lettuce (butter, romaine, green leaf, red leaf), mint, mushrooms, okra, olives, onions (all types), parsley, perilla, purslane, radishes, sauerkraut, scallions, seaweed, spinach, Swiss chard, tomatoes (if peeled and deseeded), watercress*

Dairy: *Avoid all dairy for one to three months. After that, use cheese (goat, sheep, feta), grass-fed butter, grass-fed ghee, goat milk kefir, goat milk yogurt, milk (goat or A2 milk rather than A1).*

Meat: *beef, bison, elk, lamb, moose, venison (all known to be or listed as grass fed and grass finished); chicken, duck, eggs, goose, pheasant, quail, turkey (all known to be or listed as organic and free-range, not fed soybeans); anchovies, bass, calamari, clams, crab, halibut, lobster, mussels, oysters, salmon, sardines, scallops, shrimp, tongol tuna (all known to be or listed as wild)*

Nuts and seeds: *almonds, Brazil nuts, chestnuts, coconut, flaxseeds, hazelnuts, macadamia nuts, pecans, pine nuts, pistachio, psyllium, walnuts. Note that peanuts and cashews are not nuts but legumes and cashews, which are not a nut but a seed.*

Beverages: *coffee; tea (black, green); filtered water, spring water, or sparkling water with lemon or lime wedge*

Chocolate: *low-sugar dark (72 percent or higher)*

Fat: *avocado, MCT, nut, and olive oils*

Fermented food: *kimchi, pickles, sauerkraut*

Flour: *almond, arrowroot, cassava, coconut, green banana, plantain, sweet potato flour*

Fruit: *avocado and berries (blueberries, blackberries, raspberries, strawberries). These are the best due to their low sugar content.*

Resistant starch: *green banana, green mango, green papaya, jicama, parsnips, rutabaga, sweet potato, taro root, yams, yucca*

Seasonings: *anise, basil, capers, celery seed, cinnamon, cloves, cocoa powder, cumin, curry powder, ginger, oregano, peppermint, rosemary, saffron, sage, spearmint, thyme*

Starch: *flax bread, millet bread. Add Indian basmati white rice after avoiding for at least one month, sweet potatoes, yams, cassava, carrots, taro root, yucca, jicama, tortillas (from cassava, cassava and coconut, or almond by Siete brand), and bread made from almond, coconut, or cassava, such as Julian Bakery paleo bread.*

Supplements: *prebiotics, probiotics, psyllium husk powder, and, if needed, vitamin D_3, hydrolyzed collagen, L-glutamine, magnesium, omega-3 (See appendix B.)*

Sweeteners: *Just Like Sugar (inulin), monk fruit sugar, stevia*

STARVING THE BAD

As you focus on consuming veggies, proteins, beverages, fermented food, and other food that supports the growth of good gut bacteria, you simultaneously starve the bad bacteria. This is the second part of the equation, and it only requires one simple rule: if it hurts your gut, don't put it in your body.

So how do you know what to avoid, minimize, or eliminate? The answer is to steer clear of the seven causes of a leaky gut (increased intestinal permeability): antibiotics, NSAIDs, acid-blocking meds, GMO food, chlorine in drinking water, pesticides, and intestinal infections.

Starving the bad means not putting any more of items 1–6 into your body if you can help it. The biggest hurdle for many will be the fact that they are taking medications (items 1–3), whether doctor prescribed or over-the-counter. Abruptly stopping may not be advisable, and you may need to wean off meds such as antibiotics, acid blockers, NSAIDs, and aspirin under your doctor's care or under the care of a functional medicine doctor, but your gut needs a break.

So what should you do? I don't recommend stopping medications right away. Focus on healing the gut, and let the body respond. The end goal is to add nothing to your gut that hurts it in any way. If it takes a few weeks before you can do that, then so be it. But the sooner, the better.

In addition to avoiding the seven causes of leaky gut mentioned previously, you need to remove these common enemies from your daily diet: gluten; high-sugar, high-carb, highly processed food; dairy; lectins; artificial sweeteners; emulsifiers; and saturated fats. The shift away from these common enemies of the gut is more dramatic for some people than others, but it needs to happen.

When it comes to these enemies of your gut, plan your escape this way: Go *less*, then go *low*, and finally, go *none* at all. For example, going gluten-free or lectin-free or sugar-free will not be a simple flip of a switch. It will take time to replace one food with another. Relax; don't put unnecessary pressure on yourself. Some changes may be immediate (e.g., not using artificial sweeteners), but others may take a little longer (e.g., going without dairy).

What is most important is that you are making lifelong habits of starving the bad bacteria while feeding the good bacteria. This is an ideal lifestyle, and your gut will be happy!

TAKING A TIME-OUT

Looking at the big picture of your overall health and lifestyle going forward, you recognize that the change may need to be gradual. But you do need to start somewhere. There needs to be a break with the past and a rollout of the new. This is why the new year is such a popular time to try to make healthy changes. If you can't start at the beginning of a new year, I suggest that you embark on this diet as one season ends and another one begins.

When you begin, give yourself the expectation that you are doing this for at least eight to twelve weeks (two to three months). You can do anything for just eight to twelve weeks, right? Naturally your body may love it so much that you wish to continue, but it is important that you mentally assign a window of time for your gut to heal.

Usually the gut begins to heal within one to four weeks. I've had some patients feel the benefits immediately, but most start to feel the effects about four to seven days into it. That means symptoms often begin to fade away around the end of your first week!

USE YOUR GUT POWER TOOLS

While you are busy starving the bad bacteria and feeding the good bacteria, you will also be busy creating new habits that will further benefit your gut. Five complementary habits go in perfect tandem with the food-eating/food-avoiding habits you have already started.

- **Psyllium husk fiber**—Take fiber (one-half to one teaspoon and eventually one heaping teaspoon) one to two times daily, after breakfast and dinner, in four to eight ounces of water. (See appendix B.)

- **Probiotics**—Take one to four probiotics per day or eat probiotic-rich food. (Add supplements if needed. See appendix B.)

- **Prebiotics**—Eventually take 12 grams of prebiotic supplements (add prebiotic-rich food if you can) a day. Start with much less if you have bloating or gas. Use caution if you have SIBO, SIFO, Crohn's disease, or ulcerative colitis; hold off, or start low and go slow. (Divine Health Biotics contains both probiotics and prebiotics; see appendix B.)

- **Polyphenols**—Add as many polyphenols to your daily routine as you can, especially organic olive oil.

- **Resistant starches**—These add options to your diet as they feed your good gut bacteria. Use caution if you have bloating, gas, SIBO, SIFO, Crohn's disease, or ulcerative colitis; hold off, or start low and go slow.

After eight weeks you can begin to add certain food back into your diet. For example, I recommend that you stay off cucumbers, tomatoes, eggplant, and peppers during the first eight weeks. This minimizes lectins. After a couple of months, by peeling and deseeding these vegetables, you may be able to eat them with only a slight increase in lectin exposure (since lectins are more concentrated in the seeds and skins).

It's the same with beans, which are excellent sources of protein. Pressure-cooking them for seven and a half minutes or longer after twenty-four hours of soaking (discard the water they are soaked in) will break down and remove virtually all the lectins, making them safe to eat. But during the first one to two months of your Healthy Gut Zone diet, I would recommend not eating beans at all.

In addition to watching lectins, you must always be aware of sugars (i.e., fructose in fruits), carbohydrates (i.e., in legumes), grains, saturated fats (i.e., in dairy products), and fatty cuts of meat. While your gut heals, the less sugar, carbs, and saturated fats you consume, the better. As for gluten, I recommend that most people stay off gluten, though an occasional small amount of food containing gluten will usually not hurt.

When you begin to slowly increase your food options, such as adding a new food each week, keep in mind that you will want to stay within the overall framework of starving the bad and feeding the good. That means

continuing to avoid the seven causes of a leaky gut and the common enemies of your gut. You know what those are.

When you add dairy back, start with sheep or goat milk products
or A2 dairy. For example, I enjoy some feta cheese in my Greek salad.
Choose low-fat, low-sugar goat milk that is fermented, such as goat milk
yogurt or kefir. Eventually you can add small amounts of A2 milk or two
to four ounces of low-fat A2 cheese, which is now available at some grocery stores, and rotate it every three to four days. There is also low-fat A2
yogurt and kefir.

Usually within three months you can add back in food you love, such
as Indian basmati white rice (limit to one-half cup per serving) or potatoes without the skin (where the most lectins are found). Rotate this food
as well as other high-lectin food every two to four days, and avoid any
high-lectin food that causes abdominal pain, excessive bloating, gas, or
other symptoms of leaky gut. Rotating inflammatory or high-lectin food
is a great way to still enjoy it yet limit it so it is less likely to harm the
gut. But do not add in sugary food, gluten, GMO food, or food high in
saturated fat.

Stay with it. Most people will find that their gut is healed within three
months.

THE HEALTH ZONE LIFESTYLE

This has always been about more than just a diet. It is about getting
healthy and staying healthy, and that is the result of a lifestyle more than
anything. As you expand your food list, I highly recommend eating a
Mediterranean-keto diet as a permanent lifestyle. I explain how to eat
this way in the next part of this book.

If any symptoms you eradicated from your life reoccur, then examine
what you are eating. The old "normalness" of bloating, gas, diarrhea,
nose-running, brain fog, fatigue, achy joints, and so on became a thing of
the past, and they should stay there.

You don't need inflammation of any sort. So pay attention to your gut
and adjust as needed. After several months most people find that their
food sensitivities noticeably faded away. Are those sensitivities gone forever? Perhaps, but maybe not. A healthy gut can handle the occasional

food that isn't gut friendly, but it should remain occasional and not part of a daily routine. That is why rotating certain food options that used to irritate your gut every three to four days is beneficial.

If you have an autoimmune disease, you may need to stay on this diet for a lot longer, and you may have to avoid most high-lectin food items and especially gluten. If it brings you the relief and health you want and need, I suggest that you make it your permanent lifestyle.

Many patients have told me that after they stopped having their symptoms, sickness, or disease, they intended to eat this way forever. It is a doable diet, a diet that always tries to make your gut happy.

And if your gut is happy, you are healthy. That is always the goal.

PART II

EMBRACE A MEDITERRANEAN-KETO LIFESTYLE

CHAPTER 5

KETO 2.0

ONE MAJOR REASON for many of the health problems we have now is the obesity epidemic, and it is only getting worse. In 2017, I wrote *Dr. Colbert's Keto Zone Diet* to help combat this epidemic, and it helped thousands of readers lose weight and control their appetites. But I soon began to hear that many people on a keto diet, including some of my patients, were being prescribed statin medications to lower their cholesterol. Some had even seen their cholesterol spike as much as one hundred points. And that wasn't all. Some keto dieters were complaining of joint pain, muscle aches, sinus issues, brain fog, gut issues, prediabetes, type 2 diabetes, hypertension, and occasionally even weight gain.

When I dug into the issue, I realized many people would revert to their old habits after achieving some weight loss on the keto diet. But now they were adding the foods they had come to enjoy while losing weight on the keto diet—such as butter, cream, cheese, coconut oil, and fatty meats that they ate while losing weight—with the excessive sugars, carbs, and starches in the typical American diet.

The keto diet is good, and it is still the absolute best way to lose weight, maintain a healthy metabolism, and fight sickness and disease (even cancers). But if people eventually revert back to their old eating habits—only now mixing the eating of a lot of saturated fats with the usual high-carb, starchy, sugary American diet—then the health benefits of a keto diet will begin to unravel.

Fortunately, there is a better way, what I call the Mediterranean-keto diet. This provides the benefits of a keto diet with a lifestyle that can be maintained long term. So I now recommend a simple two-step process for beating obesity and achieving a healthy weight for the long term.

Step 1: Start with a healthy keto diet to lose weight, gain health benefits, or treat or prevent sickness or disease.

Step 2: Then slide over to a healthy Mediterranean-keto lifestyle that enables you to keep the weight off, be healthy, avoid sickness and disease, and enjoy eating.

In the first three chapters of this section, we will explore what a healthy keto diet looks like—one that not only helps shed excess weight but does so without increasing inflammation and raising cholesterol. Then, in chapter 8, I will explain in detail how to transition to the Mediterranean-keto lifestyle. Finally, in chapter 9, I will explain how to get your metabolism to burn even hotter and prevent insulin resistance by incorporating intermittent fasting.

But first, I want to lay a foundation. Chances are you've heard of the keto diet. But you might have lots of questions about it. So let's dive in by answering the most common questions I am asked by patients every day.

What Is Ketosis?

Ketosis is the healthy and natural state where your body is burning fat rather than sugar for fuel. The standard high-carb American diet burns glucose, or sugar, while a low-carb keto diet burns fats as fuel. When your metabolism eventually shifts from sugar burning to fat burning, that is ketosis.

What Is a Keto Diet?

Everyone knows the typical American diet is a high-carbohydrate diet. In fact, the US dietary guidelines recommended that carbohydrates make up 45–65 percent of our calories per day.[1] That means if we eat 2,000 calories a day on average, 900–1,300 calories, or 225–325 grams, would be from carbs. No wonder we are fat!

These carbs—whether from grains, breads, corn, rice, beans, fruits, potatoes, juices, sugar, pasta, cereals, crackers, sodas, or other sources—undergo a transformation in our bodies, turning into glucose, which then becomes our primary source of fuel. Any extra glucose is stored as glycogen in our muscles and liver and as fat in the liver, abdomen, hips, thighs, and buttocks. This is simply what the body does.

As I previously mentioned, when you strategically lower your carbohydrate intake to a point where your body burns fats instead of sugars as its main fuel source, you enter a state called ketosis. Limiting your daily carb consumption is the biggest part of the equation, and that will do wonders to anyone's health, but we can't stop there. The other half of the equation is to eat healthy fats and proteins. Here's your daily macronutrient breakdown during the keto phase of your diet:

- 75 percent fats
- 20 percent proteins
- 5 percent carbs

The high-fat and moderate-protein components of the keto approach don't just improve your body's ability to efficiently utilize and burn fat stores, but they also play a pivotal role in satiety, boosting your energy levels, and reducing inflammation in the body.

As the body enters a state of ketosis, characterized by reduced glucose availability, it shifts gears to burn ketones and fats for energy. Ketones are synthesized in the liver through the breakdown of fats, and fats become the primary energy source, a process aptly named fat oxidation. This causes a remarkable shift in your metabolism—one that's centered on the use of fat reserves. It's like your body's metabolism is stoked into a blazing furnace.

Interestingly, you can burn fat even without rigorous exercise. However, incorporating gentle physical activity—think about a leisurely, twenty-to-thirty-minute walk three to five times a week—can speed up this process. That is the power and efficiency of a keto diet.

How Long Does It Take to Reach Ketosis?

For individuals in good health, ketosis typically sets in within two to seven days after you reduce carbohydrates to approximately 5–15 percent of your daily dietary intake. If you are insulin resistant, prediabetic, or diabetic, it may take longer (often four to eight weeks) to enter ketosis.

But regardless of your specific circumstances, rest assured that you will eventually reach ketosis and enjoy the many benefits of this metabolic state.

How Long Can You Stay in Ketosis?

You have the flexibility to sustain a state of ketosis for as long as you like; it's a health-conscious choice. I advise maintaining this fat-burning state until you achieve your targeted weight or successfully address any health challenges you may be contending with. Following that, consider transitioning to the Mediterranean-keto lifestyle for ongoing well-being.

Will Ketosis Burn Your Body Out Eventually?

Normally, our bodies store over 40,000 calories as fat and approximately 2,000 calories in the form of glycogen in the liver and muscles (approximately 400 calories in the liver and around 1,600 calories in the muscles). This means there's no need to worry about ketosis depleting your energy resources.[2] Furthermore, the food you eat will consistently supply your body with more fuel, allowing ketosis to continue indefinitely.

How Do You Know You Are in Ketosis?

When you are in ketosis, you are in control of your appetite, and you may feel as if you can skip a meal because you still feel satisfied many hours after your meal. When in ketosis, you usually feel satisfied, energized, and mentally focused.

So when your daily carbohydrate intake gets down to approximately 20 grams, if you feel as if you're in ketosis and have positive symptoms to match, then you're probably in ketosis. And if you're noticing weight loss, that's a further sign that you are likely in ketosis. To know for sure, you can take a test that measures the ketones present in your system.

How Do You Test for Ketosis?

When you're in a state of ketosis, your body burns fat, which is converted to ketones in your liver. These ketones are carbon compounds produced in the liver from the breakdown of fat that your body uses as energy, and they come in three distinct forms:

1. acetone (which you can measure in your breath)

2. acetoacetate (which you can measure in your urine)

3. beta-hydroxybutyrate (which you can measure in your blood)

The actual number of ketones in your body typically ranges from 0.5 to 3.0 millimolar (mM) when you are in ketosis, and you measure with a blood ketone meter (which is similar to a blood glucose meter). Interestingly, in the first month or two of being in ketosis, you can usually measure all three types of ketones (using a breathalyzer, urine test strips, and a blood test meter). However, as time goes by, only the beta-hydroxybutyrate ketone remains consistently measurable. To measure this, you'll need a blood ketone meter.

Is Ketosis Testing Required?

In a relatively short amount of time, you'll develop a sense of when you're in ketosis. But if you want to test your ketone levels as you acclimate to your keto diet, by all means, do so. I typically suggest using urine test strips at first, as they're cost-effective, user-friendly, and very effective for the first month. After that, you'll need to transition to a blood test meter. While the blood test strips are somewhat pricier than the urine test strips, they are the most accurate way to measure ketones.

Yet it's important to acknowledge that many people prefer not to meticulously track their ketones—and that's perfectly fine. If this is you, pay extra attention to your body—how you feel, your dietary choices, and so forth. You're essentially developing an internal sensitivity that enables you to recognize when you're in ketosis. This skill is invaluable and will benefit you the rest of your life.

How Long Should You Track Ketosis?

If you have cancer, obesity, sickness, or disease, I recommend that you test for ketones for the first three to six months on a keto diet. That helps, as shifting into ketosis is often a little more difficult with health-related issues. If you are healthy during the first four to six weeks of a keto diet, it is handy to be able to test (especially urine test strips) for ketones, but if you get a feel for it and don't want to test, that's fine. It's entirely up to you.

What Bumps You Out of Ketosis?

Here are five of the most common causes for people bumping themselves out of ketosis:

1. Not consuming enough fat (the goal is 75 percent)—This is often a lack of olive oil, but make sure you are getting the right amount of fats per meal per day. For a woman on 1,600 calories a day, that is 10 tablespoons of fat a day, or 3.33 tablespoons per meal. For men, it's about 15 tablespoons a day, or 5 tablespoons per meal.

2. Eating too much protein (the goal is 20 percent)—Remember, if you eat too much protein, the extra protein converts to sugar.

3. Eating too many carbs (the goal is 5 percent)—This is only 20 grams a day or equivalent to 1.5 slices of bread. It's not much, so monitor your carb intake carefully for a few days. Also, watch for those carbs that can sneak in with nut butters, artificial sweeteners, and sauces. It's best to calculate your net carbs, which is the total carbs minus the dietary fiber. For instance, a handful of almonds has 6 grams of carbs but 3.5 grams of dietary fiber; 6 grams (of total carbs) minus 3.5 grams (of dietary fiber) equals 2.5 net carbs.

4. Eating too much (practice eating until satisfied)—Dial back your total food intake by 5–10 percent. That will adjust all your macros. Chew each bite twenty to thirty times. Put your fork down between bites, and enjoy good conversation with family.

5. Unexpected stressors (be patient, ketosis will kick in)— This is often out of your control, but rest assured that ketosis will happen. Keep moving forward.

For most people, it's usually too many carbs or not enough fats. These are admittedly the two biggest changes from the standard American diet, so it is understandable that it takes some getting used to. Keep going, keep your macros in line, and your body will follow your lead.

WHAT DO YOU DO WHEN WEIGHT LOSS PLATEAUS?

Everyone hits a plateau when they are trying to lose weight. It's a universal occurrence, regardless of the diet you're following—including the keto diet. It's interesting to note that approximately 90 percent of those who embark on a keto journey do so with the intention of shedding excess weight. Yet every single individual among them inevitably encounters a weight-loss plateau along the way. This is true for every patient of mine who has embraced the keto lifestyle.

Visualizing weight loss as a flight of stairs is often helpful. As you progress, you experience periods of weight loss, followed by intervals when the pace slows or halts for a few weeks. During these times, you can either wait or make adjustments, and weight usually drops again; then it slows or stops, so you can wait or adjust again, and on and on. Losing weight on a keto diet involves making a series of incremental changes, much like stepping down a staircase. Nothing is wrong with you. You may have simply maxed out or slowed your weight loss with what you are doing. The solution lies in either continuing what you're doing on the keto diet or making modest modifications to break through the plateau.

For individuals age sixty and above, especially women, it's crucial to note that weight loss may be slower, and plateaus might last longer. Consistency is key, as the keto diet will work, just at a more gradual pace.

Should you find yourself occasionally cheating on your diet, that is OK. It's not the end of the world. It will simply slow your progress. So if you cheat, forgive yourself and move on.

Considering the average adult woman in the United States consumes around 1,600–2,400 calories in food per day, to lose weight, women should decrease their food intake to 1,600 calories per day while maintaining the macros of 75 percent fats, 5 percent carbs, and 20 percent proteins.

Adult men eat an average of 2,400–3,800 calories per day. To lose weight, men should reduce their food intake to 2,000–2,400 calories per day while maintaining the same macronutrient proportions.

When you hit a plateau, the key question is, What's the underlying cause? Then assess all the available information. Keep in mind that you haven't hit a genuine plateau until you've been in the same place for three to four weeks. Avoid pressuring yourself; it's not mandatory to lose weight every week. After three to four full weeks have passed, then you can say you've hit a plateau.

Remember the flight of stairs. On your weight loss journey, you will drop pounds, hit a plateau, drop more weight, hit a plateau, and on and on. A plateau doesn't mean you can't lose weight or the keto diet doesn't work for you. There's no need for panic. Honestly evaluate your approach, make necessary adjustments, and commit to keeping going. Ultimately, with time and determination, you will attain a weight that aligns with your desired health and sense of freedom.

How Is Ketosis a Lifestyle?

Everyone wants their bodies to be fat-burning machines. Yet committing to a strict keto diet over the long haul is a challenge not many are willing to embrace. Despite the allure of being in a constant state of fat-burning, many individuals, whether it's been a span of three months or three years, eventually gravitate back to eating lots of carbs. Unfortunately, this can yield unfavorable outcomes, particularly if the keto diet included excessive saturated fats and is followed by a high-carb regimen.

The solution lies in transitioning from the keto diet to the Mediterranean-keto lifestyle, or even alternating between the two. This shift is a seamless progression. Once the healthy keto diet has steered your body toward your desired outcomes—be it weight loss or overcoming illness—the time has come to segue into the Mediterranean-keto lifestyle.

Within the Mediterranean-keto lifestyle, the macronutrient ratios are slightly different: approximately 50–55 percent fats, 20–25 percent proteins, and 20–25 percent carbs. You can adjust these ratios to align with your unique health goals, but the beauty lies in the fact that fat tends to remain your body's primary energy source instead of sugar. This is a result of your body's natural adaptation to ketosis, causing it to evolve into an efficient fat-burning machine.

Embracing the Mediterranean-keto lifestyle—characterized by lower carb intake, generous healthy fats, and moderate protein consumption (like the keto diet with a touch more flexibility)—your body engages in cycles of entering and exiting ketosis. This dance is much like a flying fish; it lives in the ocean, yet it can glide over the waves for long distances, then land back in the water, and then zoom out again.

Throughout this process, your body will continue to burn fat as its primary fuel source. While the degree of fat utilization may vary from day to day, you control this fat-burning engine through your dietary choices. This is how ketosis can become a way of life.

Ketosis is indeed the focal point, the nucleus of wellness. On a fairly strict keto diet, your body basically stays in a state of ketosis, morning, noon, and night.

When you transition to the Mediterranean-keto lifestyle, while you continue to reap the health rewards and some of the weight loss benefits of the keto diet, your food regimen will be more relaxed. (We'll delve deeper into these specifics in the forthcoming chapters.) Ketosis is the healthiest state for your body. As a diet and then as a lifestyle, it makes perfect sense. This way of life empowers you to enjoy good health, it's adaptable, and it gives you the freedom to enjoy life to the fullest. It's exactly the place you want to be. It's where all of us want to live!

CHAPTER 6

MAJOR ON THE MACROS

WHEN DISCUSSING THE keto diet or ketosis, the word *macros* is likely to come up. Macros, a shorthand for macronutrients, encompass the three primary nutritional categories: carbohydrates, proteins, and fats—the core constituents of our daily intake. Every food contains these macros, albeit in varying proportions. Understanding and monitoring these macros lays the foundation for reaping the rewards of the Mediterranean-keto lifestyle.

In the preceding chapter I briefly addressed the manner in which we adjust these macros from the conventional Western, or American, diet to the strict keto diet, and further into a balanced keto diet, which I prefer to call the Mediterranean-keto diet. Here are those percentage distributions side by side for a clear visual comparison:

Diet	Carbs	Fats	Proteins
Typical Western diet[1]	50 percent	34 percent	16 percent
Strict keto diet	5 percent	75 percent	20 percent
Mediterranean-keto diet	20–25 percent	50–55 percent	20–25 percent

At the macro level, the two biggest changes between the conventional American diet and a strict keto diet are a considerable reduction in carbohydrate consumption and a substantial increase in the intake of healthy fats.

For most people, transitioning from a 50 percent daily carb intake to a mere 5 percent carb intake is, in itself, an effective weight loss strategy. However, it's the increase in healthy fats, the decrease in carbs to just 5 percent, and the moderate protein intake at 20 percent that work together to rev the metabolism, combat illness, and truly propel the diet into high gear.

By healthy fats, I'm talking about the fats present in sources such as olive oil; avocado oil; nuts; seeds; fish including wild salmon, sardines, mackerel, and herring; omega-3 fish oil; select grass-fed meats; turkey; chicken; specific dairy products; and more. We'll discuss each macro in this chapter, but let's begin with fats.

UNDERSTANDING FATS (MACRO 1)

At its core, the effectiveness of a keto diet hinges on your body's ability to burn fat as a healthy, clean, efficient source of energy. That is the core macro of a keto diet. If your aim is to get into ketosis to lose weight to combat sickness and disease, fats must make up approximately 70–75 percent of your daily caloric intake. This is to be complemented by a moderate amount of protein and a very low carb intake.

For those following a keto diet—or anyone striving for good health—it's crucial to focus on consuming good fats. This includes monounsaturated fats, very limited amounts of saturated fats, and the good polyunsaturated fats. Conversely, it's wise to steer clear of the bad polyunsaturated fats, trans fats, and foods fried in polyunsaturated fats, such as potato chips and french fries.

PUT GOOD FATS TO WORK FOR YOU

You can use fat to your advantage. While this claim might seem strange, it's true. Consider this: fat plays a pivotal role in regulating the hunger hormone (ghrelin). By incorporating healthy fats such as olive and avocado oil into your diet, you're using fats to curb those relentless hunger pangs. This deliberate strategy aids in weight loss—a subtle change with a big effect.

You already know the right types of fats serve as a healthful and efficient energy source for your body. Thus, maintaining a diet rich in fats—75 percent on a keto diet, and then 50 percent when you transition to the Mediterranean-keto lifestyle—keeps your metabolism running strong.

What might come as a surprise is that you can use fat to fight the nation's number one health threat: cardiovascular disease. In a large study known as the Lyon Diet Heart Study, seven thousand people already at risk of heart attack and death were given a Mediterranean-style diet enriched with olive oil and omega-3 (fish oil). Astonishingly, their risk of heart attacks and death dropped by an impressive 30 percent![2]

Another compelling reason to increase your intake of healthy fats lies in the profound impact they have on brain health. Of particular note is the brain-nourishing power of olive oil and DHA omega-3 fats. While the keto diet as a whole has exceptional benefits for brain health, it's the inclusion of beneficial fats, with olive oil and DHA omega-3 fats at the forefront, that truly feeds the brain and makes it happy. Omega-3-rich fish oil, nut oils, and avocado oil are excellent choices for supporting brain health.

The fact that brain fog often disappears shortly after beginning a keto diet can be attributed to the higher consumption of anti-inflammatory fats, notably fish oil and olive oil. These fats serve as vital nourishment for the brain, standing in stark contrast to the impact of sugars, carbs, and starches. Furthermore, the proven benefits of the keto diet extend to combating memory-related diseases such as dementia and Alzheimer's. The benefit of good fats in fighting these diseases cannot be overstated. An additional incentive to consume healthy fats is their role in facilitating the absorption of fat-soluble vitamins found in plants. Without the right fats, even eating the right plants becomes less healthy for you.

Last, it's worth noting that increased consumption of good fats has been linked to a reduction in the risk of stroke, cancer, heart disease, type 2 diabetes, and obesity.[3] These are not bad reasons for intentionally adding healthy fats to your diet, now, are they?

AVOID BAD FATS

Just as good fats help your body tremendously, so bad fats can do a lot of damage to your heart, brain, arteries, gut, energy levels, and waistline. The bad fats are

- trans fats,

- some polyunsaturated fats (e.g., oils such as soy, corn, and cottonseed),
- canola oil, a GMO monounsaturated fat, and
- excessive saturated fats (e.g., cheese and butter).

Trans fats, along with various other factors, elevate the likelihood of heart attack, heart disease, stroke, and type 2 diabetes. They also contribute to elevated levels of unfavorable low-density lipoprotein (LDL) cholesterol, escalate triglyceride levels (which contribute to arterial hardening), and reduce beneficial high-density lipoprotein (HDL) cholesterol.[4] This cascade of negative effects is, in itself, a significant source of harm.

Research has shown that excessive polyunsaturated fats can lead to elevated blood pressure, greater risk of blood clots that can trigger heart attacks and strokes, and an increase in inflammatory conditions such as cardiovascular disease, obesity, and Alzheimer's disease.[5] They also slow metabolism, increase estrogen levels, create hormonal imbalances, suppress the immune system, accelerate aging, and more.[6] Polyunsaturated fats also oxidize quickly, especially from repeated use or sunlight. These fats have been linked to increased cancer risk.[7]

When consumed alongside refined carbs or sugar, or in the absence of sufficient omega-3 levels, saturated fats can trigger inflammation. A contributing factor is our tendency to overindulge in saturated fats, particularly through dairy and meat consumption. We need only 7–10 percent saturated fats in our daily diet. Thus, it's a good idea to keep your saturated fat intake below 10 percent. One aspect of your health journey is to go through your pantry and eliminate (or donate to charity) foods that don't align with your healthy keto diet and your eventual Mediterranean-keto lifestyle.

WHEN COOKING WITH FATS

Every fat used in cooking has a smoke point, a temperature at which the fat oxidizes and causes inflammation and free radicals, so naturally you want to cook without oxidizing the fat. Because each fat has its own smoke point, each fat has a recommended use. Consider the following:

- flaxseed oil—smoke point: 107°C/225°F—drizzle, dressing
- extra-virgin olive oil—smoke point: 160°C/320°F—drizzle, sauté
- butter—smoke point: 177°C/350°F—drizzle, sauté (limited amounts)
- coconut oil—smoke point: 177°C/350°F—drizzle, sauté (limited amounts)
- macadamia nut oil—smoke point: 199°C/390°F
- almond oil—smoke point: 216°C/420°F
- ghee—smoke point: 252°C/485°F—sear, stir-fry (limited amounts)
- avocado oil—smoke point: 271°C/570°F—sear, stir-fry[8]

Making a change to your daily routine such as using the correct healthy fat is easy enough. It's knowing what is good and what is most healthy that makes all the difference. If you break fats into one group for cooking and one for adding to raw or cooked food, it would look something like this:

- for cooking: avocado oil, almond oil, macadamia nut oil (or palm kernel oil, ghee, or coconut oil, all in small amounts)

- for putting on your raw or already-cooked food: olive oil, avocado oil, walnut oil, flaxseed oil, hazelnut oil, almond oil, macadamia nut oil, cocoa butter, avocados, guacamole, unsweetened almond milk yogurt, and saturated fats, including full-fat coconut milk, grass-fed butter, grass-fed ghee, MCT oil, coconut oil, coconut meat, coconut cream, and unsweetened coconut milk yogurt, in limited amounts[9]

On a keto diet you will get most of your healthy fats from the fats you add to your raw or already-cooked food. Nuts, seeds, fish, and omega-3 supplements are also important sources of healthy fats.

UNDERSTANDING PROTEINS (MACRO 2)

The second core macro of a keto diet is the moderate consumption of healthy proteins. Alongside good fats, your body needs an adequate amount of protein to function properly.

Protein comes from a variety of sources, with each offering distinct benefits. Certain protein sources contain essential vitamins and minerals, while others come with built-in carbohydrates that can disrupt ketosis if overconsumed. Some protein options are better for when you transition to a Mediterranean-keto lifestyle, while others are hard to find or costly, making supplementation the best option in those cases.

It's imperative to bear in mind that if you consume too much protein, your body will convert the excess into glucose, thereby shifting your body's energy source back to sugar. This, obviously, undermines the effectiveness of a keto diet. The optimal target for protein intake during your keto journey is approximately 1 gram of protein per 2.2 pounds of your body weight daily.

Remember that women generally require a lower daily protein intake compared with men, typically ranging from one-third to one-half less.

Whether your aim is weight loss or with a doctor's orders getting well again, keeping your protein intake in range is key to achieving your goals.

HEALTHY PROTEINS

Each ounce of protein (e.g., egg, chicken, cheese, fish, turkey, steak, beans) on average has about 7 grams of protein in it. But as you well know, not all proteins are created equal.

Here are several healthy protein sources:

Eggs
Eggs are a superfood. They include all the amino acids that we need, all in one source. The egg yolk "is the most nutritious part—low in calories, high in protein, and full of vitamins, minerals, antioxidants, choline, and phytonutrients."[10]

People are more commonly allergic to the egg whites than the yellow yolk. If you are sensitive to either, simply rotate or use in the way that causes no problems.

The best eggs are pasture-raised eggs, which studies have shown contain two and a half times as many omega-3 fats.[11] Pasture-raised eggs can include chicken, duck, goose, ostrich, or quail.[12]

Meat

Meat in moderation, keeping to your intake per meal per day, is a good source of protein. Grass-fed meat is higher in vitamins and antioxidants than grain-fed meat.[13] Grass-fed meat has more monounsaturated fats; conjugated linoleic acid (CLA), a fat that is protective against cancer; and omega-3 fats, all of which are healthful fats.[14] If you use grass-fed meat, then you don't have to do leaner cuts, but if you don't use grass-fed meat, then choose leaner cuts (which have fewer toxins). The best sources of protein from meat include grass-fed beef, buffalo, goat, lamb, and pork; pasture-raised chicken, duck, pheasant, quail, and turkey; and wild boar, elk, rabbit, and deer.[15]

Fish

Fish are an excellent source of protein as well as necessary omega-3 (fish oil). However, for the amount of omega-3 we need per day, using supplements is a realistic option for most people.

Also, not all fish are equal. Smaller fish are less likely to have mercury, and farmed-raised fish typically have more omega-6 and less omega-3 fats from the food they are fed, and more toxins and less protein per pound. I simply recommend eating as much low-mercury wild fish as you can. One excellent reason: diets rich in wild-caught fish are associated with a 60 percent decrease in Alzheimer's.[16] The best fish to eat are wild caught or sustainably harvested, farm-raised salmon, mackerel, herring, anchovies, and sardines.[17]

Beans

Beans are a good source of protein and fiber, but they are best to avoid when on a keto diet, or eat small amounts (such as one-quarter to one-half cup) of low-starch beans (lentils, lupini, snow peas, black-eyed peas, mung beans, etc.). Later you can eat more varieties of beans and in larger amounts as part of your Mediterranean-keto lifestyle.

Why wait? A single cup of cooked pinto beans, for example, which would provide you with 12 grams of protein, would also include 35 grams of carbs! That's more than enough to stall your keto diet for the day. A small, 2-ounce piece of salmon, on the other hand, would get you the same amount of protein but with no carbs.[18]

The seldom mentioned lupini bean is high in both protein and fiber yet has very few net carbs. The starch is indigestible in your gut, so it does not make your blood-sugar levels go up and is an acceptable bean for a keto diet. [19] Until you shift to the Mediterranean-keto lifestyle, it's best to avoid higher-starch beans (such as peas, lima beans, kidney beans, baked beans, and pintos).

Soak your dried beans overnight in water with a little salt, discard the water the next morning, and then pressure-cook for at least seven and a half minutes. This soaking and cooking will help remove the lectins and decrease inflammation and gas.

If you happen to have gut dysbiosis or an autoimmune disease or are obese or diabetic, then you should eliminate beans from your diet until your gut is healthy.[20] Then you can add them in slowly and always in small amounts as long as they are soaked and then pressure-cooked for at least seven and a half minutes.

Dairy

Dairy (cheese, cream, yogurt, cottage cheese, cream cheese, etc.) is a great source of protein, but with it (as we have discussed) come a lot of saturated fats and polychlorinated biphenyls (PCBs), which are toxins. If you choose to eat dairy while on your keto diet, I recommend small amounts.

As for cheese, goat and sheep cheeses, such as feta, are lower in saturated fats, have fewer carbs, and are less likely to cause inflammation. (One of the most common food sensitivities is dairy.[21]) If you do eat cheese, use it in small amounts on your salads as a garnish.

Soy

What about soy? It has been touted as a great source of protein, but I do not recommend soy protein or soybean oil. In fact, the soy protein in fake meats, bars, and shakes is chemically altered and is a byproduct of the soybean oil production process, but non-GMO, organic, traditional soybean food, such as tofu, tempeh, miso, natto, and gluten-free soy sauce or tamari would be fine.[22]

Nuts

Nuts are a great source of protein, as well as fat, fiber, vitamins, and minerals, and they are readily available, relatively inexpensive, and usually toxin-free. They have been found to help prevent many chronic diseases (cancer, diabetes, neurodegenerative diseases, cardiovascular diseases, diabetes, etc.) and reduce blood pressure and cholesterol levels.[23]

Thankfully there are many different proteins to choose from. And when you shift from your healthy keto diet to the Mediterranean-keto lifestyle, you will have even more proteins to choose from.

Understanding Carbs (Macro 3)

The third and final fundamental component of a keto diet is to keep your carb intake low. Technically, your body requires only fat and protein, not carbohydrates, to function properly at the cellular level. This means adopting a low-carb keto diet won't kill you.

Carbohydrates are pervasive, present in nearly every food we consume. While you might enjoy the various types of carbs available, they can act as barriers between you and your health goals. Thus, it's vital that you don't allow carbs, which your body technically doesn't need, to hinder your progress.

Your Daily Carb Goal

On a keto diet your aim is to restrict your carbohydrate intake to approximately 5 percent of your overall daily consumption. Remarkably, that modest figure is almost always sufficient for fat burning for everyone, regardless of gender, age, or physical condition.

With carbohydrates kept at such low levels, the body eventually shifts from using sugar as its primary fuel source to deriving energy from fat.

This 5 percent portion of your daily intake generally corresponds to around 20 grams of net carbs per day. This will look different for each individual. Nonetheless, the ultimate objective is to keep your daily carb intake at 20 grams, sourced from healthful options. How you do it is up to you, but I recommend you get your daily carb allowance from sources such as leafy greens, nonstarchy vegetables, limited amounts of low-sugar fruits (such as berries), and nuts—all of which you need on your keto diet.

Later, when you reach your desired weight and/or accomplish your health goals and transition to the Mediterranean-keto lifestyle, you'll have the leeway to incorporate more carbs into your diet. Until then, the carbohydrate allowance is understandably more restrictive, but it's doable, especially if you keep your eyes on your ultimate goal.

A DAY IN THE LIFE

Divide your daily limit of 20 grams of healthy net carbs into the meals you eat. You'll be pleasantly surprised by how effective this approach can be. For example, for breakfast, enjoy a gently cooked over-easy egg paired with half a cup of cooked spinach sprinkled with 1 ounce of feta cheese crumbles and drizzled with 2 tablespoons of olive oil. This adds up to roughly 2 grams of net carbs.

Should your lunch consist of chicken-avocado lettuce wraps—consisting of half an avocado, a tablespoon of avocado mayo, a splash of lemon juice, 6 ounces of chicken breast, several lettuce leaves, a half cup of chopped walnuts, spices, and a drizzle of 2 tablespoons of olive oil— the net carb tally would be around 6 grams.

Furthermore, if for dinner you have salmon with asparagus—consisting of a 6-ounce salmon fillet, approximately seven asparagus spears, feta or grated Parmesan cheese, a medley of spices, and another drizzle of 2 tablespoons of olive oil—you'd be at about 4 grams of net carbs.

In short, if you were to eat three meals like these, your net carb consumption for the day would amount to a mere 12 grams, all sourced from healthful carbohydrates. Thankfully, there are a variety of delicious menu options in a keto diet that will keep your daily net carbs at 20 grams or less. (Several recipes are listed in appendix A.)

IT'S A FACT

There are many keto calculator options to choose from. This is one that I like and often recommend to my patients: https://calculo.io/keto-calculator.

Consuming more vegetables and fiber has been proved necessary and beneficial. Also watch for opportunities to eat omega-3-rich foods, as well as take omega-3 supplements.

Since your carbohydrate intake is so limited, it is imperative to make each carb choice count. Research healthy low-carb options, explore alternatives to your favorite foods, and experiment with new recipes. Prioritize low-sugar, low-starch vegetables, since vegetables—particularly salads—are a crucial component of a wholesome keto diet. You'll quickly learn which vegetables will keep you within your daily net carb quota of 20 grams and which could potentially set you back.

During the strict keto phase, read food labels carefully. Sugars are hidden in an array of products—sauces, condiments (especially ketchup), nut butters (particularly peanut butter), spices, and more—which can add carbs and undermine your daily efforts.

Ultimately, the carbs you choose will dictate the overall efficacy of your keto diet. The stringent 20-gram net carb limit serves as the optimal strategy for weight loss and the incineration of unwanted fat. It is also the key that unlocks the entire keto diet. Reducing your carb intake is the pivotal element for success on the keto diet.

Now that you better understand fats, protein, and carbs, you are more prepared not only to lose weight through a strict keto diet but also to live in the Health Zone!

CHAPTER 7

THREE WAYS TO MAKE A KETO DIET HEALTHIER

THE KETO DIET has many great health advantages that make it beneficial for everyone. Who wouldn't want to slow the aging process, shed
excess weight, get healthy, and avoid common ailments?

As a doctor, I frequently encourage my patients to adopt a healthy keto
diet. Wanting to maintain my health, manage my weight, and prevent
disease, I practice the principles I recommend.

After following the keto diet myself, I subsequently transitioned to a
Mediterranean-keto lifestyle once I reached my desired weight. This and
the next chapter will show how seamless this shift can be. These paths
converge harmoniously, with the Mediterranean-keto lifestyle evolving
organically as the next phase after the keto diet.

As you begin the keto diet journey, it is vitally important that you
avoid the pitfalls that others on a keto diet have encountered. Through
my years of using and researching the keto diet, I've seen certain gaps
that need to be filled. Among these gaps is a need for three important
additions: increased vegetable intake, increased fiber consumption, and
increased omega-3 consumption.

Despite the myriad benefits to the keto diet, these issues must be
addressed if we are to safely maximize the keto diet and transition to the
Mediterranean-keto lifestyle.

1. EAT MORE VEGGIES!

Believe it or not, on average most keto dieters fall woefully short on their
vegetable intake.[1] We all need 4–9 cups per day of low-sugar, nonstarchy

vegetables. I always recommend the low-starch, low-sugar veggies on the list (and yes, a few are technically fruits):

KETOGENIC VEGGIES

- » *artichokes*
- » *asparagus*
- » *avocados*
- » *bean sprouts*
- » *broccoli*
- » *brussels sprouts*
- » *cabbage*
- » *cauliflower*
- » *celery*
- » *garlic*
- » *greens (kale, collard, mustard)*
- » *lettuce*
- » *mushrooms*
- » *onions (of all sorts)*
- » *radishes*
- » *spaghetti squash and summer squashes such as yellow squash and zucchini (not winter squashes such as acorn, butternut, buttercup, or pumpkin, which are high in starch)*
- » *spinach*

With these vegetables, you can eat all you want! (Please choose organic whenever possible.)

Peppers and tomatoes are known to cause gut issues, so you should eat them sparingly or not at all. Carrots are fine to eat, but because of their high sugar levels, I recommend them in small amounts (a quarter cup or less). On a keto diet you always must keep in mind the number of daily carbs. If you eat too many carrots, your body will slip right out of ketosis for the day.

This rule also applies to fruit. If the sugar content is too high for you to stay in ketosis, you will simply need to consume smaller amounts or wait until you are ready to shift from a strictly keto diet to the Mediterranean-keto lifestyle, where you can eat more fruit.

2. GET MORE FIBER!

I emphasized this in chapter 3 as the primary gut power tool, and I want to reiterate its significance: you need more fiber! While many high-fiber food options might not initially align with your keto diet, they will become integral to the subsequent Mediterranean-keto lifestyle, particularly foods such as beans, peas, and lentils.

As is customary on a keto diet, you must monitor your carb intake. But no matter how much fiber you plan to consume, I always recommend taking plant fiber, specifically in the form of psyllium husk powder. Derived from the husks of *Plantago ovata* seeds, this fiber source boasts zero net carbs, and equally crucial, it's both economical and effortlessly integrated into your daily regimen. (For recommended supplements, see appendix B.)

Psyllium husk powder is the perfect blend of soluble fiber (70 percent) and insoluble fiber (30 percent). The soluble part helps you feel full, facilitates digestion, nurtures gut health, and lowers cholesterol and blood sugar, among other benefits, while the insoluble part helps ensure healthy, regular bowel movements.

If you grapple with gut-related complications or ailments, I encourage you to see chapter 3 for my guidance on gradually incorporating psyllium husk powder, beginning with a conservative intake. Once your gut is restored, I recommend integrating 1–2 tablespoons of psyllium husk powder daily: one after breakfast and the other following dinner or before bed. This regimen translates to 10 grams of fiber daily, given that each tablespoon has 5 grams of fiber. You can progressively increase your intake to ensure you get all the fiber your system needs. Your body will undoubtedly thank you.

3. Boost Your Omega-3 (Fish Oil) Intake!

I've written about the benefits of omega-3s in many of my books, but there is one newly discovered benefit of omega-3 that changes the game for keto dieters. As you know, keto diets are typically high in saturated fats. This is where omega-3 comes in. When your body is low in omega-3, these saturated fats cause inflammation.[2]

I'm not saying to boost your levels of omega-3 so you can maintain an excessive saturated fat intake. Not at all. My point is, almost everyone on a keto diet consumes some saturated fat, and if you are not also getting enough omega-3 in your diet, you are letting inflammation in.

Conventional recommendations are typically a minimum of at least 500 milligrams of omega-3 daily. Yet, considering how desperately your body needs omega-3, I suggest doubling that to at least 1,000 milligrams daily. (Personally, I take 2,000 milligrams twice daily.)

For many of us, the only way to get this much omega-3 fat is through a dietary supplement. Virtually all health food and grocery stores offer a variety of omega-3 fish oil options. Opt for omega-3 that contains more eicosapentaenoic acid (EPA) than docosahexaenoic acid (DHA), such as 700 milligrams of EPA and 300 milligrams of DHA, or as close to a 2:1 ratio as you can get since a 2:1 EPA-to-DHA ratio appears to be particularly effective in addressing inflammatory risk factors.[3] If you want to improve brain function, I recommend a fish oil with a higher concentration of DHA and less EPA, or around a 1:1 ratio of EPA to DHA.

The American Heart Association recommends that people with coronary heart disease consume 1,000 milligrams of a combination of EPA and DHA each day.[4] The European Food Safety Authority states that omega-3 supplements can be safely consumed by adults at doses up to 5,000 milligrams per day.[5] From now on, don't let your body run short of omega-3.

And there you have it: three significant gaps that often exist within a typical keto diet. I would venture to say that only a fraction of keto dieters are getting enough of these crucial additions. The significance of these additions cannot be overstated. Integrate them into your daily routine, for now and the future. Embrace these changes, and you'll undoubtedly reap the benefits!

CHAPTER 8

A HEALTH ZONE FUSION: THE MEDITERRANEAN-KETO APPROACH

I T'S TIME TO establish your healthy keto diet framework so you can dive in and begin the process. Because there is much to remember, this chapter is intentionally designed to be clear-cut and systematic. As a quick reminder, these are the fundamental macronutrient levels essential for a stringent keto diet:

- 75 percent fats
- 20 percent proteins
- 5 percent carbs

Everything is founded on this cornerstone. When you are ready to transition to the Mediterranean-keto lifestyle, every aspect will build on those macronutrient values.

Essentially, you are on a journey from where you are to where you desire to be—a progression from point A to point B. Your health objectives will be your inspiration to keep going.

Step-by-step, this is where your keto diet begins:

STEP 1: DEFINE YOUR STARTING POINT

To establish your starting point, begin by weighing yourself and capturing photos and body measurements. Record this information in a journal, on your phone, or in whatever way suits you best. While initially it might not seem important to define this starting point, it will indeed become a valuable source of information as you progress. Moreover, it can serve as a source of encouragement as you begin to lose weight, drop inches, and see other positive changes.

STEP 2: DO THE MATH

Reduce your overall daily food consumption by roughly 20 percent, keeping within your designated macronutrient ratios (75 percent fats, 20 percent proteins, 5 percent carbs). Calculate the calories per macro, and then convert these calories into grams per macro.

For women

In the United States, the typical adult woman consumes around 1,600–2,400 calories daily. For weight loss purposes, you'll want to reduce this to 1,600 calories per day while maintaining your healthy keto diet macros. (Usually, a 20 percent reduction in daily food intake is effective for weight loss, making 1,600 calories a solid starting point.) Following the macro ratios and 1,600-calorie target, this equates to 1,200 calories from fats, 320 calories from proteins, and 80 calories from carbs.

For men

In the United States, the typical adult male consumes around 2,400–3,800 calories each day. For weight loss, it's recommended to reduce your daily caloric intake to 2,000–2,400 calories while maintaining your healthy keto diet macros. (A 20 percent reduction in daily food intake is generally effective for weight loss, making 2,000–2,400 calories per day an excellent starting point.) With the macro ratios and 2,400-calorie target, this translates to 1,800 calories from fats, 480 calories from proteins, and 120 calories from carbs.

According to the USDA, the calorie-to-gram ratios are 9 calories per 1 gram of fat, 4 calories per 1 gram of protein, and 4 calories per 1 gram of carbs. Calculating for women at 1,600 calories per day, this equals 133 grams of fats, 80 grams of proteins, and 20 grams of carbs. For men at 2,400 calories per day, this amounts to 200 grams of fats, 120 grams of proteins, and 30 grams of carbs. (I still generally recommend starting men on 20 grams of carbs.)

Many people don't know how many calories they consume each day. To establish a baseline, track your calories for a day or two. Or you can simply choose a starting point (e.g., 1,600 calories for women, 2,000–2,400 calories for men) and start there. This approach generally works for most people.

For people who are obese or have a larger body size, I usually recommend they start by reducing their daily intake by 20 percent for a period of two to four weeks. Afterward, they can decrease it by another 20 percent, gradually working their way down to the target of 1,600 calories for women or 2,000 to 2,400 calories for men. This approach allows for more gradual and sustainable weight loss.

Ultimately, you decide how many calories to consume each day. Whatever number you choose as your starting point, begin there.

STEP 3: APPROXIMATE YOUR FOOD

Calculate the macro quantities of each meal. For women following a 1,600-calorie plan and consuming three meals a day, this translates to roughly 44 grams of fats per meal (equivalent to around 3.33 tablespoons of fats per meal), 27 grams of proteins per meal (approximating 4 ounces of proteins per meal), and 7 grams of carbs per meal.

For men consuming 2,400 calories a day spread out over three meals, this means approximately 67 grams of fats per meal (about 5 tablespoons of fats per meal), 40 grams of proteins per meal (around 6 ounces of proteins per meal), and 10 grams of carbs per meal (or 7 grams per meal if you opt for 20 grams of carbs per day).

If your starting daily caloric intake differs from these examples, that's OK. Just make sure you know your daily target and divide it by your intended number of meals per day. For most individuals, I would suggest beginning with three meals a day, and later on, you can explore intermittent fasting, which I'll delve into in chapter 9.

Once you've established the approximate grams of each macro per meal, it's time to put it into practice. Begin to practice figuring out the macros (fats, proteins, and carbs) with healthy foods and using that information per meal.

Fortunately, lists containing the macronutrient values of various foods are readily available online, as are numerous keto-friendly recipes. I've also included some healthy keto recipes in appendix A to help you get started.

THE FUSION OF KETO AND MEDITERRANEAN

I previously mentioned that in a strict keto diet, aimed at weight loss or combating illness, the food breakdown is generally 75 percent fats, 20 percent proteins, and 5 percent carbs. However, the more flexible Mediterranean-keto lifestyle shifts to 50–55 percent fats, 20–25 percent proteins, and 20–25 percent carbs.

What makes the Mediterranean lifestyle keto is that because of the foods the people eat, the olive oil consumption, the salads, the veggies, and the macronutrient proportions, their bodies drift in and out of ketosis. They get the benefits of a healthy keto diet without really having to do anything extra! They don't have to go on a diet as we do—it's their way of life. It's the presence of extra-virgin olive oil bottles on their tables; the consumption of healthy, wild, fresh foods; their coffee, tea, and (for some) red wine habits; and the incorporation of omega-3 and fiber in their diet. Their lifestyle steers clear of heavily processed foods, high-sugar and high-carb diets, and sedentary living. It's not eating highly processed foods, not living on a high-sugar and high-carb diet, and not living a sedentary life.

It's a lot of good things that collectively form their way of life, and that's our goal as well. The foods you choose to eat in the Mediterranean-keto lifestyle will likely cause you to experience ketosis more often than those solely eating Mediterranean foods.

In my experience, once your body adapts to being in ketosis, you can increase your carb intake to around 50–75 grams per day (and even up to 100 grams for some) while still maintaining ketosis. This is one reason beginning with a healthy keto diet before transitioning to the

Mediterranean-keto lifestyle is recommended. However, the choice is always yours.

TYPICAL MEDITERRANEAN FOOD

» *Olive oil and other healthy fats*

» *Vegetables (fresh salads and sautéed veggies)*

» *Meats (seafood, poultry, goat, sheep, and cow)*

» *Fresh herbs*

» *Beans, peas, lentils, and hummus*

» *Lower-carb fruits (raspberries, blueberries, blackberries, strawberries, etc.)*

» *Nuts and seeds*

» *Yogurt and kefir*

» *Eggs*

» *Dark chocolate*

» *Coffee, black tea, and water*

» *Red wine (in moderation: one glass per day, or best, not at all)*

If your starting point is the Mediterranean-keto lifestyle, I recommend you aim for a daily intake of 50 grams of carbs, particularly during the initial months when your body is adjusting to relying on fat as its primary source of energy instead of sugar. Gradually, you can raise your carb intake to 75–100 grams daily, and in certain cases, even up to 125 grams per day. This is still much lower than what the typical American consumes, which is 250–500 grams of carbs per day.

THE BASICS OF THE MEDITERRANEAN-KETO LIFESTYLE

The Mediterranean-keto lifestyle differs from a conventional Mediterranean diet in terms of carb content. Not everything labeled as Mediterranean aligns with this lifestyle, just as not all keto diets are equally healthy. The key is to select nutritious foods that suit your goals and consume them in appropriate proportions.

At its core, the Mediterranean-keto lifestyle entails consuming ample healthy fats, moderate amounts of quality protein, lots of vegetables and salads, and limited amounts of good carbs. This way of living avoids or limits packaged and processed foods, dairy, artificial sweeteners, high-carb and high-sugar items, and unhealthy fats.

How does this translate into real meals? You'll find Mediterranean-keto lifestyle recipes in appendix A, yet the specifics can vary from person to person. Remember, the macro distribution of 50–55 percent fats, 20–25 percent proteins, and 20–25 percent carbs serves as your foundation. Your individual metrics, health objectives, and whether you're aiming for weight loss or maintenance will influence how these macros are divided.

If you're concerned about how to balance these macronutrients, refer back to chapter 6 for a comprehensive breakdown. The Mediterranean-keto lifestyle, characterized by a healthful Mediterranean diet low in sugars and carbs, is profoundly beneficial. Eating that way has a proven track record that will encourage and perhaps even amaze you.

Undoubtedly, olive oil plays a pivotal role in the Mediterranean-keto lifestyle, just as it does in a healthy keto diet. What's remarkable and comforting is that Mediterranean cuisine, enriched by olive oil, correlates with reduced rates of cancer.[1] In fact, for over twenty years, nineteen different studies tracked more than thirty-five thousand people and found that olive oil use was directly linked to lower cancer risks.[2] And for women specifically, those who stuck with a Mediterranean diet and all of its extra-virgin olive oil had a much lower level of breast cancer risk than the normal population.[3]

Beans, peas, and lentils are also a very important component of the Mediterranean-keto lifestyle (in moderation) if you have no gut issues. They are packed with protein, vitamins, minerals, and fiber and help control blood sugar while blocking disease-causing oxidation.[4] They also have some starch (which counts as a sugar) and lectins, which are inflammatory compounds.[5] But removing the lectins is easy enough. As I mentioned earlier, you simply soak the beans overnight in water with a little salt and discard the water the next morning. Then you pressure-cook them for at least seven and a half minutes. The soaking and cooking process removes almost all the lectins, thereby decreasing inflammation.

Other healthy carbs include, but are not limited to, such food as sweet potatoes, yams, cassava, and taro root, usually limited to the size of a tennis ball, or half a cup per serving.

If you want a lifestyle that keeps you healthy, charges your metabolism so you can lose weight, and helps protect you from countless sicknesses and diseases, I cannot recommend anything better than the Mediterranean-keto lifestyle.

The Danger of Lectins

Lectins, which are large proteins found in plants, are heavily concentrated in leaves and seeds of all plants. They also appear in animals that consume these plants. High concentrations of lectins are found in grains, particularly wheat, as well as legumes (such as beans, soybeans, peas, and lentils) and nightshades (such as tomatoes, potatoes, peppers, and eggplants). These lectins can often trigger inflammation in the gut and potentially throughout the body.

Lectins attach themselves to sugar molecules like sialic acid, which are found in various areas including the gut, joints, and brain. This binding can result in inflammation, leading to issues such as brain fog, joint pain, gut disturbances, and more. Additionally, lectins frequently contribute to weight gain. Corn and brown rice contain lectins too, although white rice has notably fewer. One particularly troublesome lectin is wheat germ agglutinin (WGA), present in wheat bran. WGA, found in whole wheat products such as bread and pasta, behaves similarly to insulin, promoting weight gain and possibly fostering insulin resistance. In many cases, today's wheat can be extremely inflammatory for numerous individuals. Wheat can produce 23,788 different proteins,[6] and any of these have the potential of triggering inflammation. However, most inflammation from wheat is caused by two specific gluten proteins: glutenin and gliadin.

The typical Mediterranean diet often includes a lot of wheat products and other carbs that can lead to inflammation. Due to this, I suggest incorporating low-lectin carbs in moderation, along with low-carb fruits at around 50–100 grams per day. If you're dealing with gut issues,

I recommend reading my book *Dr. Colbert's Healthy Gut Zone* before beginning the Mediterranean-keto lifestyle.

Farmers have long known that pigs and cattle tend to gain weight mainly from consuming corn and soybeans rather than grass or hay. Wheat, corn, and soy are all rich in lectins and are prevalent in many processed foods.

When following the Mediterranean-keto lifestyle, it's advisable to avoid most high-lectin foods and starches. Instead, opt for beans, peas, or lentils that have been soaked and pressure-cooked for approximately seven and a half minutes to eliminate most of the lectins. Other low-lectin carb choices include sweet potatoes, yams, cassava, jicama, taro root, yucca, and millet bread.

Incorporating one or two servings of low-carb fruits such as berries, plums, kiwi, citrus fruits, cantaloupe, and watermelon can also be beneficial within your Mediterranean-keto routine. Remember, you don't have to include a starch with every meal. Personally, I often include a starch at dinner to aid in sleep and to maintain my weight (I tend to lose weight easily). However, many individuals prefer to have a single fruit serving with two daily meals in the Mediterranean-keto lifestyle and one starch a day once they've achieved their weight goal.

The USDA recommends that the average adult consumes two cups of fruit per day, but it's wise to opt for low-carb fruits to help maintain your weight.

STARTING YOUR MEDITERRANEAN-KETO LIFESTYLE

Similar to beginning the keto diet, when you're ready to start your Mediterranean-keto lifestyle, there are a few steps you should take. If you've already been on a healthy keto diet, these steps might come naturally to you.

If you're transitioning to the Mediterranean-keto lifestyle from a healthy keto diet, incorporating additional carbs (such as beans, peas, lentils, hummus, sweet potatoes, low-sugar fruits, and other wholesome carb sources) will likely be a welcomed adjustment.

Following are the three essential steps everyone starting the Mediterranean-keto lifestyle should take.

STEP 1: ESTIMATE YOUR CALORIES

Start by calculating your daily caloric intake using the macro proportions of the Mediterranean-keto lifestyle: 50–55 percent fats, 20–25 percent proteins, and 20–25 percent carbs.

The specifics may differ for men and women, and they can even vary from person to person. Given that each individual's body is unique, the following breakdown is a general guideline that suits most people. As you become more attuned to your body's needs and see your health improve, you'll likely identify whether your body needs more or less of a specific nutrient.

For women

The average adult woman in the United States consumes around 1,600–2,400 calories per day. To lose weight, you want to decrease that to 1,600 calories per day while maintaining the Mediterranean-keto lifestyle macro levels. Based on calories per day, that means 800 calories from fats, 400 calories from proteins, and 400 calories from carbs.

For men

The average adult male in the United States consumes around 2,400–3,800 calories in food per day. To lose weight, you should decrease your food intake to 2,400 calories per day while maintaining the Mediterranean-keto lifestyle macro levels. Based on 2,400 calories per day, that means 1,200 calories from fats, 600 calories from proteins, and 600 calories from carbs.

STEP 2: ESTIMATE YOUR GRAMS

Once you have determined your calorie requirements for each macronutrient, you can convert those calories into grams. As per the USDA guidelines, the calorie-to-gram ratios are 9 calories per 1 gram of fat, 4 calories per 1 gram of protein, and 4 calories per 1 gram of carbs.

For women consuming 1,600 calories daily, this translates to approximately 89 grams of fats (equivalent to about 6.6 tablespoons of fats), 100 grams of proteins (approximately 14.3 ounces of proteins), and 100 grams of carbs.

For men with a daily intake of 2,400 calories, this results in about 133 grams of fats (around 10 tablespoons of fats), 150 grams of proteins (approximately 21.4 ounces of proteins), and 150 grams of carbs.

For individuals, whether male or female, aiming to lose weight or maintain their current weight, it's advisable to slightly reduce carb intake. I recommend around 75 grams of carbs for women and 100 grams for men.

It's worth noting that the lower your carb intake, the longer your body will remain in ketosis, which is the state where fat burning primarily occurs. If you're going straight to the Mediterranean-keto lifestyle, tracking your daily caloric intake initially can help you stay on track as you adjust to a specific caloric/gram goal per day. This aids in meal planning, making it a crucial aspect of your journey.

STEP 3: ESTIMATE YOUR GRAMS PER MEAL

For women eating 1,600 calories over three meals per day, the macronutrient breakdown is approximately 30 grams fats per meal (2.2 tablespoons per meal), 33 grams proteins per meal (4.8 ounces per meal), and 33 grams carbs per meal. (I recommend 25 grams per meal initially to lose weight and then slightly more carbs to maintain weight.)

For men eating 2,400 calories over three meals per day, the macronutrient breakdown is approximately 44 grams fats per meal (3.3 tablespoons per meal), 50 grams proteins per meal (7.1 ounces per meal), 50 grams carbs per meal. (I recommend 33 grams or less per meal initially to lose weight and then slightly more carbs to maintain weight.)

Now that you know the macronutrient targets for your Mediterranean-keto lifestyle, you are ready to begin. Thankfully, all the math and calculations per macro and recipes have already been figured out. You don't have to do it all!

You can easily find out (from books, online, apps, etc.) what the macronutrients are per food item you choose, and fortunately, you don't have to build your entire recipe list on your own (unless you want to). Use the many recipes in appendix A or at Dr.Colbert.com to begin. In time, you'll have a long list of your favorites, and you may even develop some recipes of your own!

CHAPTER 9

THE POWER OF INTERMITTENT FASTING

WHAT IS INTERMITTENT fasting, exactly? To put it simply, intermittent fasting is refraining from eating for a brief period of time.

You might have unintentionally experienced fasting before. Situations such as high-pressure work assignments or unforeseen travel may have disrupted your usual eating routine, resulting in a longer period without food than usual.

For many people, eating continues until bedtime and resumes as soon as they wake up. However, the six to eight hours of sleep at night doesn't provide sufficient time for the body to register it as a fasting period.

If the window of time without food is extended enough, your body starts perceiving it as a fasting period. This doesn't necessarily need to be twenty-four hours, three days, three weeks, or even thirty days for your body to reap the advantages of fasting.

And this is where intermittent fasting steps in. Various versions of intermittent fasting have gained popularity in recent years. Patients visiting my clinics may have experimented with several of these methods, including the following well-known approaches:

- 12/12 plan: Eat during twelve hours of your day, and fast for twelve hours.

- 16/8 plan: Eat during eight hours of your day, and fast for sixteen hours. (This is my favorite.)

- 20/4 plan: Eat during four hours of your day, and fast for twenty hours.

- 5/2 plan (also called the 5:2 diet): Reduce your food intake to around five hundred calories twice a week, on two noncon-secutive days.

- Alternate-day plan: Eat no food for one day, eat normally the next day, fast again, eat again, and so on.

Given the variety of intermittent fasting options, the assumption is that you'll consume regular (and ideally healthy) meals when you're not fasting. It's also assumed that you'll stay well-hydrated by consuming at least two quarts of clean, pure alkaline water during your fasting inter-vals. Maintaining proper hydration is of utmost importance. You can also enjoy beverages such as coffee, tea, or other calorie-free options during your fasting periods, prepared with zero-calorie natural sweeteners such as stevia or monk fruit if desired.

IT'S A FACT

Intermittent fasting can help lower blood pressure, eventually reducing the amount of needed blood pressure medication with its unpleasant side effects (brain fog, fatigue, erectile dysfunction, sluggishness, etc.). Intermittent fasting has helped hundreds of my patients with their blood pressure issues.

Moreover, it's assumed that a significant portion of your non-eating time corresponds with sleep. For instance, in the widely used 16/8 plan, individuals fast for sixteen hours, which could conveniently include eight hours of sleep. During the remaining eight hours, they abstain from con-suming food. For example, someone might finish dinner at 5:00 p.m. and not have breakfast until 9:00 the next morning. (Of course, they can still enjoy their morning coffee with only stevia.)

Alternatively, they might choose to skip either breakfast or dinner to achieve the sixteen-hour fasting goal. This two-meal-a-day approach substantially reduces calorie intake, which some find preferable and is a strategy I personally endorse.

I once had a patient who had successfully shed weight with my Mediterranean-keto diet, but she felt her progress had plateaued. By incorporating a sixteen-hour daily fast and skipping breakfast, she saw additional fat loss. Those extra fasting hours helped her achieve the desired results.

As I've said, of the various intermittent fasting options available, I prefer the 16/8 plan. Why? Because it aligns well with most patients' daily routines, increasing the likelihood they'll stick with it. Any healthy habit you can seamlessly integrate into regular life tends to yield long-term success. The 16/8 plan is an approach that's accessible to everyone, but the choice is yours. Some prefer the 14/10 plan, fasting for fourteen hours a night, which also helps. Choose the fasting plan that suits you best and commit to it so you can reap and retain the benefits.

BENEFITS OF INTERMITTENT FASTING

Numerous health advantages come from incorporating intermittent fasting into your lifestyle. In all honesty, the benefits of intermittent fasting need to be substantial because abstaining from food isn't exactly fun! Here are the top four benefits of intermittent fasting:

1. It helps you lose weight.

2. It usually improves your brain function and mental clarity.

3. It improves insulin resistance and usually lowers fasting blood sugar, insulin levels, and hemoglobin A1c.

4. It usually boosts your energy levels.

These advantages complement the array of benefits we explored earlier. The fact that our bodies can access these advantages by simply adjusting our eating routine is remarkable.

Traditionally, many medical professionals, including myself, advised patients to eat three meals a day, with particular emphasis on breakfast as the most important meal of the day. However, with the latest research, we've come to understand that it's healthier to skip either breakfast or dinner and opt for a two-meal-a-day approach.

Thanks to intermittent fasting, the guidelines have evolved. Some people begin by fasting once a week and gradually progress to incorporating it for three to seven days a week.

Benefit 1: weight loss

When we eat, a significant portion of what we consume is converted into glucose and stored as glycogen. Typically, our bodies store enough glycogen from our meals to sustain us for about twelve hours.

This doesn't mean we won't experience hunger if we abstain from eating; rather, it means our bodies continue to use sugar as an energy source during those initial twelve hours. If we don't consume more food within that timeframe, our metabolism shifts, and we begin using fat as our primary fuel.

Unless we extend the fasting period beyond twelve hours, our bodies tend to remain in the mode of burning sugar. To access the fat-burning state, we merely need to extend the fasting period between meals. Naturally, burning fat results in weight loss.

This explains why some people opt for plans like the 16/8 method or even the 4/20 strategy, in which twenty hours of fasting translate to around eight hours of fat burning. Since most people burn fat within sixteen hours of fasting, the 16/8 plan is also effective, and many people can do this for several days each week.

Certain studies suggest that the transition from sugar burning to fat burning can occur after fasting for as little as eight to twelve hours.[1] However, I prefer to be conservative in fat burning, so I recommend fasting for at least twelve hours.

Consistently following your chosen fasting plan, week after week and month after month, will help you lose weight. When your body is burning fat every day, even if it's only in small increments, the impact over time can be significant.

Several years ago, the *Molecular and Cellular Endocrinology* journal compared the results of forty different intermittent fasting studies and concluded that intermittent fasting works for losing weight.[2] You would expect as much, but forty studies is conclusive.

I've observed that some patients prefer a traditional weight-loss approach where they reduce their daily calorie intake. However, a growing group of patients are finding intermittent fasting more manageable on a daily basis. They don't need to meticulously count calories or purchase specific foods; they simply regulate their eating patterns.

Once more, the weight-loss strategy you choose is completely up to you.

As a side note, the shift from burning sugars to fats also benefits your heart. Triglyceride fats are consumed during the fat-burning process, directly lowering the risk of cardiovascular disease![3] Intermittent fasting has been shown to also lower blood pressure.[4]

Benefit 2: improved brain function

Given the rising prevalence of cognitive disorders, it's important to carefully consider anything that can boost your brain health.

As a healthcare professional, I'm witnessing a growing influx of patients grappling with conditions such as dementia, Alzheimer's, Parkinson's, and various other neurological issues. The fact that intermittent fasting has been shown to reduce the risk of many neurological disorders means that everyone should pay close attention to intermittent fasting.[5]

If it helps you and your loved ones and is admittedly easy to do, then what's the holdup?

Johns Hopkins School of Medicine professor Mark Mattson has done decades of research on the connection between what we eat and how our brain functions. In regard to fasting and intermittent fasting, his research has found that fasting can do the following:

- help the brain ward off Alzheimer's and Parkinson's
- improve memory and mood
- protect neurons against plaque buildup[6]

In addition, David Perlmutter, MD, boldly states, "In the absence of calories, life-sustaining, protective genes responsible for cellular repair and protection are activated, inflammation is reduced, and anti-oxidative defenses are increased. This means that simply going without food for a while may have anti-aging, anti-inflammatory, and anti-tumor benefits that are available to anyone, at any time."[7]

As we've previously discussed, once you've fasted for approximately twelve hours, your body usually transitions from burning sugars to using fat as its energy source. During this process, ketones, which are fatty acids, are released into the bloodstream. These ketones play a crucial role in weight loss.

What's more, these same ketones play a vital role in preserving your brain function, and we all want that! They even provide some protection from neurodegenerative disorders, Alzheimer's disease, and seizures.[8]

As an advocate of preventive medicine, I strongly believe it's important to treat an issue before it escalates into a significant problem. Many patients who visit my practice are noticing a gradual decline in their cognitive functions. Neurological challenges rarely arise suddenly; they often develop over time.

If you can put ketones to work as a preventive measure through intermittent fasting, then do it! I have seen this yield remarkable results. Some patients' cognitive abilities have improved within just a few weeks of incorporating fasting. One study found it took only six weeks for their focus group (older adults who all suffered from mild cognitive impairment) to see memory improvement after increasing their ketone levels.[9] In fact, intermittent fasting and the ketones that work their way to your brain as a result have been found to even help new nerve cells grow in your brain.[10]

On a deeper level, the release of ketones as a result of fasting also stimulates the production of a protein known as brain-derived neurotrophic factor (BDNF). What exactly does this BDNF protein do? It "strengthens neural connections, particularly in areas involved in memory and learning"![11] In addition, BDNF has been found to help protect our brains from Alzheimer's and Parkinson's disease.[12] Interestingly, BDNF levels can be boosted in more ways than one. Physical exercise and mental tasks will do it, as will reducing your caloric intake through fasting.[13]

Again, if there's something that benefits our brain health, it's in our best interest to do it. Taking a preventive approach to our brain health is far wiser than waiting until the situation becomes critical. The fact that intermittent fasting, and fasting in general, has been found to play a significant role in helping to stop, slow down, or even reverse neurodegenerative conditions such as Alzheimer's, Huntington's, and Parkinson's diseases should be ample motivation to take action today![14]

Benefit 3: improved insulin resistance

Reducing insulin resistance through intermittent fasting might not initially strike you as important, but understanding what insulin resistance is might change your perspective.

People dealing with type 2 diabetes or prediabetes already know how important insulin is. Yet insulin isn't relevant only to those with diabetes. In fact, the very reason people have type 2 diabetes is because their bodies have become insulin resistant.

Here's what is happening: Higher and higher levels of insulin in the bloodstream are needed to bind to the insulin receptors on cell surfaces, enabling glucose to enter cells. However, like a rusty lock, these insulin receptors don't always function efficiently. Although the key (insulin) fits the lock, it doesn't turn smoothly; considerable effort and multiple attempts with other keys (more insulin) are needed before the lock finally opens.

Figuratively speaking, intermittent fasting cleans the rust from these locks, enabling insulin receptors to accept insulin (the key) and thereby making the whole process work much more effectively. What you want is a clean lock and a single key (lower insulin levels). It's efficient, fast, smooth, and good for your body.

Insulin is essential for everyone, whether they have diabetes or not. We all require insulin to survive. The less insulin needed for the sugar-to-cell transfer, the better off you are.

So how does intermittent fasting help reverse insulin resistance?

First, being overweight or obese is a major cause of people developing type 2 diabetes.[15] The fact that approximately 30.7 percent of adults in the United States are overweight and another 42.4 percent are obese, according to the National Institute of Diabetes and Digestive and Kidney Diseases,[16] means insulin resistance is important to more people than we might think—and these obesity and overweight rates are going up year after year.

If hurting the body isn't enough, diabetes also hurts the pocketbook. According to the American Diabetes Association, as of 2017, the yearly cost of treating diabetes in the United States was about $327 billion, which included medical care and lost productivity.[17]

Once again, this cost is calculated annually, and the situation is only getting worse.

The obesity epidemic is propelling the diabetes epidemic, and it all has to do with insulin resistance. This is because each additional pound makes cellular functioning just a little more challenging.

Men, if you have a waist measurement around the navel that is over forty inches, you're likely insulin resistant. Similarly, women with a waist measurement around the navel over thirty-five inches are also probably insulin resistant. Insulin resistance commonly leads to prediabetes, and prolonged prediabetic conditions often lead to type 2 diabetes.

Insulin plays a crucial role for everyone because it allows cells to take in sugar. But if your body develops resistance to insulin, it becomes more difficult for sugar to enter the cells. To overcome this, your pancreas releases more and more insulin, hoping to improve the situation. Over time, this results in sugar lingering in your bloodstream, unable to penetrate cells. This makes you thirsty and causes frequent urination, classic indications of diabetes. This is how increasing insulin resistance leads to elevated blood sugar levels, which usually signals the approach of prediabetes or type 2 diabetes.

Left unchecked or ineffectively managed over extended periods, insulin resistance can inflict permanent harm on the pancreas' beta cells (responsible for insulin production), resulting in the need for insulin injections and other complications.

The silver lining is that it is possible to reverse type 2 diabetes! I have helped numerous patients reverse and fix their type 2 diabetes. And intermittent fasting can play an important role in helping to keep your cells sensitive to the insulin your body produces.[18]

As a whole, intermittent fasting reduces the risk of type 2 diabetes because of weight loss and less insulin resistance.[19]

The weight gain/insulin resistance battle is always connected. For that very reason, intermittent fasting is recommended for those at risk of diabetes.[20] And if you are already type 2 diabetic, I recommend it all the more.

Many people wonder whether weight loss lessens insulin resistance, or if less insulin resistance causes weight loss. The answer is yes because it works both ways, though the greatest positive change is a direct result of weight loss.

The correlation between the surge in type 2 diabetes (among other conditions) and the obesity epidemic is widely known. Consequently, shedding excess weight will naturally help curb the prevalence of these diseases.

While it may seem obvious, if you are not eating, your body doesn't need to produce as much insulin, and your insulin levels drop. After roughly twelve hours of fasting, the body runs out of stored glycogen (sugar) to burn as energy and shifts to burning fat, producing ketones, which help you lose weight. During this time of fasting, the decreased insulin levels may in turn cause the cells to release and therefore burn their stored sugars (glycogen) as energy.[21]

The faster sugars are used up, the faster the body transitions to burning fat for energy, thus highlighting the role of reduced insulin resistance in boosting weight loss.

Over the years, I've helped thousands of people with type 2 diabetes and prediabetes to reverse their symptoms, with some cutting their hemoglobin A1c levels in half. Through the healthy keto and Mediterranean-keto diets, intermittent fasting, exercise, hormone treatment (which we will discuss in part 3), and supplements (where applicable), these patients have achieved medication-free lifestyles, weight loss, and a restoration of their overall health.

For those who have struggled with type 2 diabetes for over fifteen years, reversing insulin resistance is more challenging due to the damage to the pancreatic beta cells. Nevertheless, the marked improvements and numerous health benefits of intermittent fasting still make a remarkable impact on those suffering from type 2 diabetes.

Benefit 4: boosted energy levels

Intermittent fasting also initiates a phenomenon known as autophagy within our bodies. This process involves the systematic elimination of aged cells, denatured or damaged proteins, and accumulated cellular waste. Essentially, it's like a thorough house cleaning, ridding your system of much of the cellular clutter.

However, autophagy does more than tidy up. By clearing out aging cells and removing abnormal proteins, the mitochondria present within each cell are also being cleansed.[22] In your cells, it is the mitochondria's job to produce adenosine triphosphate (ATP), which is your body's energy currency.

It's interesting to note that your heart muscle has more mitochondria than any other muscle in your body because your heart is constantly pumping. Additionally, your skeletal muscles and liver also have substantial amounts of mitochondria. But stored fat tissue contains relatively few mitochondria because it undergoes so little metabolic activity.[23]

When the mitochondria are cleaned of abnormal proteins and cellular trash, this revitalization process causes improved mitochondrial function—and that translates into more energy for your body![24]

It's much like a flowering bush that has been neglected. Once you prune away the dead flowers, leaves, and stems, the bush blooms. Fresh flowers appear, and the plant regains its health and vitality.

The reason for cleansing the mitochondria is quite similar. Think of it as maintenance for aging. The aging process impacts us all, coupled with the effects of free radicals and diseases that exacerbate mitochondrial damage.

As we grow older, our mitochondria suffer wear and tear, accumulating cellular waste. This gradual accumulation slows down our production of ATP, the energy currency of our bodies.

This decline becomes painfully apparent when you compare the energetic, vibrant demeanor of young patients who visit my office to the complaints of patients in their sixties, seventies, or eighties. Energy production tends to decrease with each passing decade. I have seen patients at age sixty who drag into my office. After seventy, their energy is usually even lower, and after eighty, they often have hardly any energy left at all.

It all boils down to mitochondria struggling to meet the body's energy demands.

Recently, I encountered a patient in his midseventies, slightly overweight, on multiple energy-sapping medications, and engaged in missionary work abroad. He was so discouraged he wanted to quit doing the work he loved, which was teaching, preaching, and ministering. After introducing him to the keto diet and recommending intermittent fasting just one day a week, he said it sounded so easy he could probably do that every day. Within a few months on this regimen, his energy rebounded. He now feels youthful, and his active travel schedule attests to the fact that it's working.

Intermittent fasting helps clear away cellular damage, which then helps repair and restore damaged mitochondria. That boosts the production of ATP, giving you increased energy, vitality, and stamina.[25]

Talking About Food

Recommendations for what to consume during an intermittent fast varies widely. Some say when you're not fasting to eat whatever you'd usually eat. Certain plans permit specific snacks during fasting, while others suggest sticking to water or noncaloric beverages only, and this is what I recommend. Some skip breakfast or dinner, while others fit three meals within a smaller window of time. Still others prefer a more traditional approach to fasting, going days without eating.

You get to choose whatever fasting plan you prefer.

You also get to choose what you will eat. I recommend following the 16/8 approach and eating the delicious foods detailed in parts 1 and 2 of this book, just within an eight-hour window. In my personal experience while fasting, coffee sweetened only with stevia and no creamer makes for a great breakfast (one can have an MCT oil powder when the fast is broken), followed by homemade soups for lunch and dinner that incorporate healthy fats/oils.

For a midday boost, snacks such as celery stalks with almond butter, avocado, carrots, and so on, with nuts are great to help me get through the day. I like to drink jasmine green tea and sunset cinnamon tea with stevia during my intermittent fasting. I call it my brain-boosting and energy-boosting tea. Some patients call it their fat-burning tea.

The Power of Intermittent Fasting Is Yours

Intermittent fasting presents a remarkable opportunity to access the many advantages of fasting. Despite being partial fasting, it works wonders. Incorporating it into your lifestyle can yield incredible results. Who wouldn't want to lose weight, improve cognitive function, improve insulin resistance, and boost energy?

Nearly every patient who walks into my office is grappling with a condition, ailment, or symptom that is directly tied to one of those four issues. Not only do they want these benefits; they *need* them for their long-term health.

For those with symptoms or a family history of conditions such as Parkinson's, Alzheimer's, dementia, or age-related memory decline, intermittent fasting can be a powerful ally. A patient of mine, a real estate agent, had to leave his job because mild dementia left him in a constant brain fog, causing him to make unfortunate mix-ups during property viewings.

While he adopted a healthy keto diet and optimized his testosterone levels, it was intermittent fasting that truly gave him the mental clarity he sought. Within just six weeks of practicing intermittent fasting, his mental fog lifted, and his sharpness of mind returned. He happily returned to his real estate career.

Seize the opportunity intermittent fasting presents, and put it to work in your life. You'll be glad you did.

PART III
MAKE A GREAT LIFE WITH HORMONE OPTIMIZATION

CHAPTER 10

CRACK THE CODE OF HORMONE HARMONY

FOR MANY YEARS in my practice, when patients came to me with symptoms such as brain fog, mild depression, and increasingly cold hands and feet, one of my first responses was to balance their hormones, being careful not to push any hormone level too high. The problem was that their long list of symptoms didn't always go away. In time I came to understand that it wasn't enough just to balance a person's hormones; we usually needed to optimize them.

After attending advanced hormone training by some of the top antiaging experts, gynecologists, and hormone doctors in the world, I learned how to detect suboptimal hormone levels, treat the various hormones in the best possible way, and optimize hormone levels to the point where patients are usually able to regain their health.

The difference it has made in my patients' lives has been nothing short of amazing! I could tell stories for hours—of young women who could not get pregnant, much less carry their babies to term, who now have one or more children of their own; of aging men who were able to rebuild muscle; of women who were able to get completely off their antidepressant medications; of women who escaped the nightmare of migraines, weight gain, irritability, anxiety, or premenstrual syndrome (PMS); and men and women who no longer suffer from high blood pressure, insomnia, high cholesterol, type 2 diabetes, fibromyalgia, chronic fatigue, or chronic pain. And it was mainly because we were able to optimize their hormone levels.

WHAT ARE YOUR SYMPTOMS?

Symptoms, whether good or bad, are usually a reflection or echo of what is already happening inside our bodies. Everything we eat, drink,

81

breathe, touch, experience, believe, and choose to do *today* will be reflected in our bodies *tomorrow* and in the days to come. That means the symptoms you have today are the result of the many yesterdays that led up to this point. It also means that doing something different today will bring about a different tomorrow as well!

Is this not exactly the principle from Scripture of sowing and reaping?

> For whatever a man sows, that he will also reap.
> —GALATIANS 6:7

This always holds true. It is a fact of life. Thankfully, when we sow good seeds, we also reap good rewards in return.

So what are your symptoms? Every doctor visit begins there. But what do the symptoms mean? And is there something you can really do about your persistent symptoms? If you have suffered from recurring symptoms, you are desperate for answers. I have met people who have put on a brave face and soldiered through ten, twenty, thirty, even forty years of some pretty discouraging symptoms. Years! Without real answers, the symptoms will persist. But do you really want to wait that long before you get help?

Below is an alphabetized list of hormone-related symptoms and diseases I see every single day. Every doctor does. These may also be the very symptoms you are dealing with right now. Maybe you are looking for help, trying to find answers, and getting increasingly frustrated at how hard it is to break free.

Take a few minutes to look through this list. As you do, rate the degree that the symptoms affect you. The list and the rating system will help bring clarity to your own unique situation. Later in the book we will explore these hormone-related issues and what you can do about them.

Absence of morning erection	Autoimmune disease
Absence of zest for life	Belly fat
Achy joints	Bladder infection/leak
Acne as an adult	Bone loss
Alzheimer's	Brain fog
Arthritis	Brittle nails

Carpal tunnel syndrome

Cellulite

Chronic infections

Cold backside

Cold hands/feet

Cold intolerance

Concentration difficulty

Constipation

Dementia

Depression

Diabetes (type 2)

Dizziness

Dry eyes

Dry skin

Enlarged prostate

Erectile dysfunction

Excessive earwax

Exhaustion

Facial hair increase

Fatigue

Fatty clavicles

Fibromyalgia

Fluid retention

Food cravings

Forgetfulness

Frailty

Frequent illness

Frequent naps

Frequent UTIs

Goiter

Grumpiness

Hair breakage or loss

Hard/round stools

Heart disease

Heart palpitations

Heavy periods

High blood pressure

High cholesterol

High cortisol levels

High insulin levels

Hoarse, husky voice

Hypoglycemia

IBS

Infertility

Infrequent sexual climax

Insomnia

Irritability

Lack of sex drive

Light-headedness

Loss of curves

Loss of energy

Loss of enjoyment

Loss of stamina

Low body temperature

Lupus

Man boobs

Migraines	Sagging breasts
Miscarriages	Salt craving
Mood swings	Sarcopenia
Muscle loss	Scleroderma
Muscle pain	Skin wrinkles
Muscle weakness	Slow metabolism
Nausea	Strokes
Nervousness	Sweating
Obesity	Sweet craving
Osteoporosis	Swollen jawline
Panic attacks	Thinning eyebrows
Parkinson's	Thinning skin
Poor memory	Tremors
Prediabetes	Turned down lip corners
Puffy/bags under eyes	Vaginal dryness
Ridged nails	Weight gain
Ringing in the ears	Worse allergies

How Hormones Get Out of Sync

While a minority of my patients experience hormonal imbalances due to genetic factors, the overwhelming majority can attribute their hormonal issues to these factors:

- age (Hormones such as estrogen, progesterone, testosterone, DHEA, pregnenolone, and growth hormone gradually decline as we age, especially after age fifty.)

- obesity (associated with low testosterone levels and higher estrogen levels in men)

- diet (Meats including red meat and poultry, dairy, and eggs all contain estrogen. Beef fat and chicken fat from the United States contain much more estrogen than lean meats. US beef contains much higher levels of estrogen than Japanese beef.[1] Soy contains plant estrogen—isoflavones—that has weak estrogenic activity. And regularly consuming trans fats from processed foods and many desserts lowers testosterone levels.)

- insulin resistance (type 2 diabetes, prediabetes, obesity). If a man has type 2 diabetes, he is twice as likely to have low testosterone as a man without diabetes.

- medications [Many drugs can lower testosterone levels, such as cholesterol-lowering statin drugs; SSRIs including fluoxetine (Prozac), paroxetine (Paxil), and citalopram (Celexa); and opioids. Antihypertensive meds including beta blockers, ACE inhibitors, and spironolactone also lower testosterone levels, and antihistamines such as Benadryl can interfere with the production of testosterone in the testicles.]

- chronic illness or insomnia (usually associated with lower testosterone levels)

- sedentary lifestyle

- inadequate sleep

- excessive stress (causes the body to release cortisol, and chronically elevated cortisol can inhibit testosterone production in men)

- the cumulative effect of marijuana (can increase estrogen production and decrease testosterone levels in men)

- hormone disruptors (Reduced testosterone levels and increased estrogen levels can be attributed to the presence of parabens and phthalates. These chemicals are commonly found in various personal care items, including shampoos, conditioners, moisturizers, hair care products, shaving creams, and gels. Parabens function as preservatives, preventing the growth of bacteria and mold, and are also used as fragrance ingredients in numerous personal care products and cosmetics. Meanwhile, phthalates serve as softening agents in items like shampoos, conditioners, and cosmetics.)

- endocrine disruptors [These substances can also elevate estrogen levels and hinder thyroid function. They encompass Bisphenol A, perchlorate (a byproduct of aerospace and weapons industries found in certain US drinking water sources), dioxins, PCBs, polybrominated diphenyl ethers (PBDEs), which are utilized in flame retardants, per- and polyfluoroalkyl substances (PFAS), which are used in nonstick pans, and many others. For additional details, refer to *Dr. Colbert's Hormone Health Zone*.]

- pesticides (Many pesticides are xenoestrogens, or chemicals that behave like estrogen. Organochlorine pesticides have significant estrogen-mimicking potential. Since the 1970s, dichlorodiphenyltrichloroethane (DDT) and other common organochlorine pesticides have been banned in the United States and the European Union. However, they are still manufactured and used in developing countries. These pesticides are mainly found in the food animals eat and are then stored in the animals' fat. They are usually present in fatty meats, cheese, butter, and cream.)[2]

These variables have a direct impact on hormone levels, and it's evident that none of them are linked to your genetic makeup. In a sense, this is good news because it implies that you have the power to influence your hormones by the choices you make rather than being bound by predetermined factors. However, it's possible that your past choices haven't always been health-focused, which can lead to negative consequences for your body and brain down the line. The really good news is that your body is generally resilient and can often recover when you make the necessary adjustments.

Even more encouraging is that as we prioritize the health of our body and brain, they respond positively. This is something everyone can appreciate. Your blood test results offer valuable insights into your hormone levels and can help you determine the areas that may need attention.

I've covered hormones extensively in my book *Dr. Colbert's Hormone Health Zone*, exploring how to achieve balance and optimization. For most people, simply following the guidance outlined in part 3 of this book will help significantly in rebalancing hormones and thus lead to a healthy life.

The healthy living principles presented in all my Zone books are interconnected. This means that while you focus on restoring gut health, adopting a healthful Mediterranean-keto diet, practicing intermittent fasting, and optimizing your hormones, you are simultaneously engaging in activities that can prevent, decelerate, manage, halt, or even reverse Alzheimer's and dementia.

Yes, what you just read is indeed accurate—that's how our bodies operate.

HORMONES AND BRAIN HEALTH

Your brain reaps substantial benefits from having the correct hormones in optimal quantities. This underscores the importance of maintaining balanced hormones, particularly when it comes to brain health.

On a cellular level, hormones, which act as key chemical messengers, are released by different glands throughout your body and directly enter your bloodstream. Subsequently, these hormones journey to every corner of your body to carry out their designated functions.

The hormones that exert the most significant influence on your brain include

- cortisol (helps your brain focus and respond in a time of stress, but too much cortisol harms neurons, especially in the hippocampus),

- pregnenolone (helps memory and protects neurons),

- testosterone (helps neurons survive and thrive),

- DHEA (helps decrease the effects of stress), and

- estrogen (for women, it improves the brain's nerve cell connections and helps the brain's blood flow, and yes, estrogen is also important for the male brain, but not in excessive amounts). (See chapters 13 and 14.)

If these hormones are not at the right levels, your brain and body pay a big price!

Too much cortisol: This typically stems from chronic stress and can lead to a decrease in the uptake of glucose (the fuel supply for the brain), especially in the hippocampus, the region of the brain responsible for memory creation and storage. Eventually this causes impairment in short-term memory and the depletion of neurons in this area of the brain. If you suspect chronic stress, consider measuring your saliva's cortisol levels at 8:00 a.m., noon, 4:00 p.m., and 8:00 p.m. It's worth noting that drawing blood through venipuncture can elevate cortisol levels, making a salivary test a more accurate method for measurement.

Not enough pregnenolone: Once more, it's important to highlight that chronic stress is detrimental to the brain. Pregnenolone—a compound the body uses to synthesize estrogen, testosterone, DHEA, and cortisol—illustrates this effect. Unfortunately, during periods of heightened stress, pregnenolone is directed toward cortisol production, diverting it away from the creation of other brain-protective hormones like testosterone, estradiol, and DHEA.[3] The consequence of decreased pregnenolone levels includes cognitive decline and even weight gain, among other effects. The presence of chronic stress and elevated cortisol levels can lead to the shrinkage of the prefrontal cortex and the hippocampus, two pivotal regions responsible for memory and learning processes. Pregnenolone is naturally synthesized in the adrenal glands, women's ovaries, and men's testes, with its levels decreasing as individuals age.

A neurohormone, pregnenolone has the potential to reduce the risk of dementia and support the growth and survival of neurons within the brain. Notably, individuals with Alzheimer's and dementia tend to have lower pregnenolone and pregnenolone-derived neurohormone levels in the key areas of the brain associated with memory.[4] Because pregnenolone is used as a precursor for essential steroid hormones like testosterone, estradiol, and DHEA, an increase in cortisol levels due to chronic or acute stress will result in a decreased availability of pregnenolone for the production of these hormones.[5] I recommend micronized pregnenolone, which can be purchased at a health food store or online. I typically recommend 25–50 milligrams one to two times per day, and I monitor patients' pregnenolone levels. See appendix B.

Not enough testosterone: Both men and women have and need testosterone. While men have approximately ten times more testosterone than women, low testosterone levels increase the Alzheimer's and dementia risk for both genders. Testosterone is important because of all the benefits and protection it should provide for your brain: helping memory, preventing shrinkage of neurons, repairing neurons, improving blood flow, and decreasing your risk of Alzheimer's and dementia. But if your testosterone levels are low, then all this is most likely not happening.

TARGET HORMONE LEVELS

Please note that the following hormone target values differ from what I provided in my book Dr. Colbert's Healthy Hormone Zone. With the knowledge I now have, I feel these are the best hormone levels for the brain. I have also lowered estrogen and raised TSH values due to the high incidence of breast cancer (one in eight women[6]). With all that in mind, here are my recommended hormone-level targets:

» *estradiol 20–50 pg/mL for women over fifty (some women may need higher levels) and 20–40 pg/mL for men (with ideal levels being 20–30 pg/mL)*

» *FSH 23–50 IU/L for women over fifty*

- » progesterone 1–20 ng/mL
- » pregnenolone 100–250 ng/dL
- » cortisol (AM) 10–18 mcg/dL
- » DHEA sulfate level for women 100–350 mcg/dL
- » DHEA sulfate level for men 150–500 mcg/dL
- » total testosterone men 500–1000 ng/dL
- » free testosterone men 15–26 pg/mL
- » total testosterone women 50–150 ng/dL (and even higher to 200 ng/dL for those female patients with osteoporosis or sarcopenia)
- » free T3 3.0–4.2 pg/mL
- » reverse T3 <20 ng/dL
- » TSH <2.0 mIU/L
- » anti-TPO negative

Not enough BDNF: Brain-derived neurotrophic factor (BDNF) aids in strengthening the synapses within your brain. Low levels of testosterone and estradiol hormones also lead to decreased BDNF levels, which in turn contribute to the accumulation of amyloid plaque![7]

Not enough DHEA: Testosterone, pregnenolone, and DHEA, a steroid known for safeguarding brain neurons, are among the most effective treatments for traumatic brain injuries such as concussions. DHEA has neuroprotective effects on the brain. As people age, their DHEA levels decrease, rendering the brain more susceptible to harmful chemical and metabolic influences. Additionally, chronic stress contributes to the depletion of DHEA levels, as evidenced by a study showing significantly reduced DHEA levels in stressed individuals compared to those without stress.[8] I usually start most women on 10 milligrams of micronized DHEA, taken one to two times per day, and 25 milligrams for men, taken once or twice daily.

Not enough estrogen: Estrogen is known to improve nerve cell connections and blood flow in the brain. It is also known to help protect against memory loss and prevent Alzheimer's.[9] It's common to need estrogen supplements after menopause, and they offer valuable defense against Alzheimer's and dementia. Many patients often benefit from a mild to moderate increase in estrogen levels, which can lead to improved brain function. To protect against breast cancer, I recommend adding a dose of 150 milligrams of diindolylmethane (DIM, derived from broccoli) to the regimen once or twice a day. Sufficient estrogen decreases the risk of Alzheimer's in women by up to 50 percent![10] Women need to have a normal mammogram before starting estrogen and need to have annual mammograms.

Estradiol (estrogen) is also essential for men. After the age of fifty, many men experience elevated estradiol levels due to the conversion of testosterone into estrogen, a process known as aromatization. To counteract this, I place men on DIM at a dosage of 150 milligrams once or twice daily, which helps reduce estradiol levels. In many cases, increased belly fat leads to higher estrogen levels, as belly fat produces estrogen and many inflammatory compounds.

More and more men are being placed on weekly testosterone injections by their physicians, and many of these men have high estradiol levels due to the aromatization of testosterone to estradiol. This can lead to breast tissue formation, erectile dysfunction, and increased fat in the hips and thighs. Optimizing testosterone levels has significantly improved memory in many men, and this often results in optimized estradiol levels, as some of the testosterone converts into estradiol. For more detailed information, you can refer to my book *The Hormone Health Zone*.

Having balanced thyroid hormone levels is another key factor in good brain function. Hypothyroidism, characterized by an elevated TSH level in lab tests, is associated with a heightened risk of dementia. For every six-month period during which TSH remains elevated, the risk of dementia increases by 12 percent.[11] However, when properly balanced, it can lead to improved cognitive performance. Many patients have reported a lifting of brain fog, greater mental clarity, and improved memory after starting natural desiccated thyroid hormone. Restoring optimal brain function is always a welcome outcome! I treat most patients with suboptimal thyroid function with natural desiccated thyroid, such as NP Thyroid.

If your hormone levels have been low and you are working to bring them up and balance them, I suggest you check your hormone numbers every three to six months until your hormone levels are balanced or optimized, then check them again every six months. That will give you a very accurate picture of where you are and how you are progressing.

Getting DHEA, pregnenolone, testosterone, estradiol, and free T3 (thyroid) levels balanced or optimized is usually enough to help protect the brain from memory loss, high cortisol levels, and chronic stress. If someone has Alzheimer's or dementia, regardless of what stage they might be at (mild, moderate, or severe), balancing or optimizing their hormones will usually be beneficial.

Every effort to balance your hormones will usually help support and strengthen your brain, making it more difficult for amyloid plaque to build up. That is always the goal when it comes to preventing, slowing, managing, stopping, or reversing Alzheimer's and dementia.

How to Balance Your Hormones

Hormone levels, for both men and women, typically begin to drop around age fifty. That's normal, but no excuse, for there is much that we can do to improve our hormone levels and keep them balanced. The healthy protection from balanced hormones is an absolute must-have!

The best place to begin in your effort to balance your hormones is with an overall plan of good health. That is because balanced hormones usually mirror a balanced life.

Based on the thousands of patients I've seen over the years, I would say the best way to guarantee your hormones remain balanced would be to

- have an active lifestyle;

- eat healthy (especially a healthy keto or Mediterranean-keto diet);

- live a low-stress lifestyle;

- exercise regularly;

- correct insulin resistance;

- get seven to eight hours of good, restful, well-oxygenated sleep;

- take few or no medications, except Viagra, which may reduce your risk of Alzheimer's by 70 percent;

- take nutritional supplements;

- fix (not bandage) anything chronic in your life; and

- avoid the ten dementogens: (1) heavy metals such as mercury, arsenic, and lead; (2) environmentally acquired illnesses such as Lyme disease and those acquired from mold; (3) anticholinergic medications, including some antihistamines and drugs used to treat allergies, depression, and GI disorders (see *Dr. Colbert's Healthy Brain Zone* for a list); (4) too much copper; (5) artificial sweeteners and sugars; (6) alcohol; (7) trans fats; (8) general anesthesia, the effects of which can be minimized; (9) marijuana and other drugs; (10) and chronic infections such as Lyme disease, cold sores, chronic bronchitis, and chronic sinusitis. I go into detail about each of these dementogens in *Dr. Colbert's Healthy Brain Zone*.

This list will help balance and may eventually boost many people's hormones. However, with advancing age, most people will eventually need bioidentical hormone replacement therapy.

Every effort taken to help balance your hormone levels is an equal step forward that often can turn off or turn down whatever is damaging your brain and turn on all the good things that build up your brain such as brain-derived neurotrophic factor (BDNF), which restores the brain.

It's all good, and it all counts. Keep it up!

Do I Need to Optimize My Hormones?

For most people, balancing and boosting their hormone levels is enough to get their health back on track and to prevent, slow, manage, stop, or reverse Alzheimer's and dementia. For a more comprehensive understanding of hormone optimization, you can delve into *Dr. Colbert's Healthy Hormone Zone.*

Optimizing your hormones isn't a silver bullet on its own. It should go hand in hand with maintaining a healthy diet, regular exercise, adequate sleep, stress management, and other positive habits. However, the synergy of combining these beneficial choices and practices with optimized hormones can lead to remarkable outcomes. In some instances, I've seen symptoms vanish and illnesses stop progressing and even reverse completely.

Optimizing your hormones is a crucial step toward living in the Health Zone. Balanced hormones are essential for your body and brain to effectively combat Alzheimer's and dementia. In the following chapters, we will look at ways to optimize the hormones that most commonly get out of sync, namely the thyroid, adrenal glands, testosterone, progesterone, and estrogen.

CHAPTER 11

THYROID TO THE RESCUE

WHEN WE THINK of hormones, the thyroid may not immediately come to mind. But it is a key hormone that, along with cortisol from the adrenal glands and testosterone from the sex hormones, plays a vital role in replenishing the body's energy levels. These are among several other endocrine (hormone-producing) glands, including the hypothalamus, pancreas, ovaries, testes, pineal gland, pituitary gland, and parathyroid gland.

These endocrine glands secrete hormones directly into the bloodstream, underscoring the importance of the application method (injections, patches, creams, pellets, and sublingual tablets) for achieving optimal hormone levels.

Of all the glands, the pituitary gland runs the show. It releases thyroid-stimulating hormone (TSH), which prompts the thyroid gland to generate sufficient amounts of thyroid hormones. The thyroid knows when it has produced enough thyroid hormones to meet the demands of the brain and body, and it relays this information back to the pituitary gland. This feedback loop is a fundamental component of your body's health.

These thyroid hormones control the efficiency and speed at which all the cells in your body work.[1] They are incredibly important, sensitive, and complicated, with everything taking place at the cellular level. If there is any miscommunication between the glands and hormones, it is usually reflected in how you feel. That is usually where hormone issues begin.

DEALING WITH SYMPTOMS

Doctors agree on what the thyroid does (regulates heartbeat, manages metabolism, warms you, helps grow hair/nails, restores cells, helps you sleep, and more). They disagree, however, on what to do when symptoms arise.

For historical context, thyroid problems are not a recent development. In the 1930s, it was estimated that a significant 40 percent of the entire population experienced thyroid-related concerns![2] And today? As many as 40 percent of Americans are hypothyroid (when the thyroid is not producing enough thyroid hormone).[3] I would say that about 50 percent of the US adult population has suboptimal or low normal thyroid levels, but with all the endocrine disruptors today—including BPA (bisphenol A) found in plastics and the lining of metal cans, mercury, and the common weed killer atrazine—it may be closer to 60 percent. You would think that after almost a century of medical advances we would have made some headway!

Compounding the situation is the fact that we're discussing percentages when it comes to individuals facing thyroid issues. When we factor in other hormones, the percentage of people dealing with hormone-related problems rises even higher. Drawing from my thirty-five years of medical practice, I've observed that a significant portion of patients who present with medical concerns also grapple with hormone imbalances to varying degrees.

Addressing symptoms without addressing the underlying cause is far from a solution. In most cases, this approach tends to exacerbate the situation over time, leading to a cycle of worsening conditions. Unless the root cause of the hormone imbalance is addressed, the symptoms are likely to persist, often resulting in a decline in overall health.

TESTING YOUR THYROID LEVELS

Before you schedule a blood work appointment, I recommend you test yourself at home using the basal body temperature test. Dr. Broda Barnes, a renowned thyroid specialist, used this simple test on his patients with remarkable accuracy.

For several days, measure your body temperature (placing the thermometer under your arm) each morning before getting out of bed. A typical body temperature falls around 97.8–98.2°F. If your average reading from several mornings is below 97.8°F, your body is running cold. This suggests a sluggish metabolism, which is a clear indicator of hypothy-roidism or less-than-optimal thyroid function.

When it comes to testing your blood, there are several tests you should have, including the following:

- T4
- free T3
- free T4 (optional)
- TSH
- reverse T3 (rT3)

If your body is attacking your thyroid gland (autoimmunity), such as with Hashimoto's, you will have elevated antibodies, so I also recommend testing TPOAbs (thyroid peroxidase antibodies) and/or TgAbs (anti-thyroglobulin antibodies). If your doctor won't run these tests for you, find a doctor who will. (See appendix B.) Why is getting the right test so important? Because the choice of lab tests and their erroneous normal ranges are the biggest culprit to keeping patients undiagnosed and undertreated![4]

Addressing your thyroid levels requires a solution, not just a temporary fix. Therefore, if you are experiencing symptoms of low thyroid function, such as fatigue, weight gain, cold sensitivity, dry skin and hair, brain fog, and mood changes, keep seeking answers until you find them.

When discussing the need for thyroid testing, most physicians will typically conduct the thyroid-stimulating hormone (TSH) test. Some might also check your free T4 levels. However, for an accurate picture of your thyroid function, all five tests are necessary. The TSH test is consid-ered the gold standard for thyroid testing among endocrinologists and most doctors. Nonetheless, there are critical details about this test that you need to be aware of.

Fact: TSH Measures Your Pituitary

The TSH test does assess your thyroid-stimulating hormone levels, but this hormone is primarily produced by the pituitary gland. It doesn't directly reflect cellular activity within your body but rather indicates pitu-itary function. While the TSH test may identify a fraction of individuals with low thyroid function, the results for most people tend to fall within the "normal" range. In cases where results show as "normal," healthcare professionals might prescribe antidepressants or other medications.

Dr. Mark Starr, author of *Hypothyroidism Type 2: The Epidemic,* went so far as to say, "There is no scientific evidence to support the doctors' claim that the TSH test detects hypothyroidism on the vast majority of patients."[5]

FACT: TSH LACKS INFORMATION

Regrettably, the TSH test doesn't provide enough information. Even if you're grappling with multiple symptoms, your numbers might fall within the acceptable range, masking hypothyroidism. This is a source of frustration for millions of people each year.

According to LabCorp, the standard TSH range for adults is 0.45–4.5 µIU/mL (micro–international units per milliliter). However, based on my experience, if your TSH level is over 2.0, you're likely experiencing some suboptimal thyroid symptoms. Because of the lack of information, you might be dealing with numerous symptoms yet still be diagnosed with normal thyroid function.

Optimizing thyroid levels will usually reverse the symptoms, but your TSH score may go down to 0.1 µIU/L or lower. That in turn will trigger a red flag with virtually every endocrinologist, and you may be labeled in a "hyperthyroid" state, but that is false. This "below lab range" TSH score is routinely encountered when you are optimally treated with natural thyroid medication.[6]

Optimizing thyroid levels will not induce hyperthyroidism. While many doctors might misinterpret the TSH lab results to suggest otherwise, this actually underscores the main point. Achieving optimized T3 levels (using natural desiccated thyroid) will typically lead to a decrease in TSH without triggering hyperthyroidism.

A patient of mine was persuaded by a doctor to discontinue the optimization treatment due to concerns about atrial fibrillation, stroke, heart attack, or osteoporosis. Unfortunately, upon quitting, she quickly saw her symptoms return.

Notions such as "it will weaken your bones," "it may cause fractures," or "it could lead to a heart attack or stroke" are outdated lies. However, patients must choose between feeling great and conquering their symptoms or settling for mediocrity and battling symptoms indefinitely.

Here's the solution: If your TSH levels fall below the normal range but you're feeling good, check your free T3 level. If those numbers are in range, it indicates you aren't experiencing hyperthyroidism, contrary to what some doctors and endocrinologists might assume.

Now, if your free T3 levels are really high and your heart rate exceeds 100, or you're experiencing excessive sweating or palpitations, then it's advisable to lower the dosage. Instances of this nature are exceedingly rare. Usually the free T3 levels remain within range and your body feels great. Make sure your resting heart rate stays below 100, preferably below 90.

TOTAL VS. FREE

The thyroid hormones T3 and T4 each have two forms— free and total—and there are different tests to measure each one. In both cases the test for free measures only the thyroid hormone in your body that is available and not bound by proteins, rendering it unable to be used. The test for total measures all of that hormone, whether free or protein bound (unusable). Measuring for free will give the best picture of your thyroid.

FACT: TSH DOES NOT MEASURE THE ACTIVE THYROID HORMONE

For many individuals facing thyroid-related problems, the underlying issue often is insufficient production of free T3—the active thyroid hormone that carries out significant tasks within your cells. If your TSH score is high (indicating low thyroid function), most doctors will likely prescribe a synthetic thyroid hormone such as Synthroid, or levothyroxine, comprising only T4 to normalize (lower) your TSH. I know it's confusing, but a high TSH indicates low thyroid function.

Nevertheless, the real issue lies not with T4, but rather with free T3 because it is not bound by proteins and can readily enter all cells. A substantial number of people with hypothyroid symptoms struggle to convert T4 into T3 effectively. Therefore, introducing more T4 medication into the equation usually does not resolve the issue. While some individuals may benefit from increased T4 medication, many will find their symptoms persisting. Although the T4 medication often restores the TSH lab value to a normal range, it typically falls short in addressing the array of symptoms associated with low thyroid function.

That is because TSH is a pituitary hormone and not a thyroid hormone. When the thyroid is diseased by Hashimoto's thyroiditis or is low functioning and not producing enough thyroid hormones, TSH levels will usually rise. It's like the pituitary is screaming at the thyroid, *"Make more thyroid hormone!"*

The thyroid gland then produces more T4 (thyroxine), but T4 is an inactive hormone that needs to be converted to T3 (the active thyroid hormone). T3 must be unbound from proteins to become free T3, thereby enabling it to access all cells.

Most doctors rely on the TSH test (keep in mind that the normal range for LabCorp is 0.45–4.5 µIU/mL). A TSH above 4.5 suggests low thyroid function, while a TSH below 0.45 indicates hyperthyroidism. Unfortunately, this leaves countless patients with low or suboptimal thyroid function untreated.

Once again, a significantly more accurate evaluation involves measuring the free T3 level. I recommend optimizing this level to fall within 3.0–4.2 pg/mL, or sometimes slightly higher. Optimizing free T3, the active thyroid form, typically alleviates most low thyroid symptoms. It's possible to have a normal T4 (the inactive thyroid hormone) and very low free T3 levels, yet still exhibit a "normal" TSH level. The TSH test often fails to identify individuals with low, sluggish, or suboptimal thyroid function.

It's clear that the TSH test falls short in offering a comprehensive diagnosis of thyroid issues. So what does the TSH test reveal? It tests your pituitary hormone within the thyroid-pituitary-hypothalamic loop, indicating whether your pituitary gland functions properly. While this insight is valuable, it does not address your other thyroid-related concerns.

SYNTHETIC THYROID TO THE RESCUE?

Synthroid was created in the 1950s to combat the ever-growing thyroid problem stemming from iodine deficiency, which affects about 40 percent of the global population.[7] It became, and still is, one of the most prescribed medications in the United States. Every year, healthcare providers write almost 100 million prescriptions for medications like Synthroid.[8]

When Synthroid came on the scene, natural desiccated thyroid (NDT) was widely used. So the creators of Synthroid commissioned a researcher to demonstrate its superiority over NDT. Surprisingly, the researcher's findings contradicted their intentions, showing NDT to be more effective. However, the company blocked her story and tried to undermine her credibility. Yet over time the reality emerged: NDT proved to be more effective than Synthroid.[9]

One of the key reasons NDT outperforms the synthetic Synthroid is its alignment with your body's natural 1-to-4 ratio of T3 to T4. In contrast, Synthroid consists solely of inactive T4.

To illustrate what is happening on the cellular level with T4 and T3, picture a skilled grandfather who has a knack for building birdhouses. They are colorful and unique and come in various sizes and colors. Yet instead of placing them outdoors to welcome birds, he stacks them up in his garage, then fills the attic and rooms, eventually leaving no space for another birdhouse.

The crucial step would be to take those birdhouses outside and allow them to serve their purpose by housing birds. The active element—the essence that defines a birdhouse—is missing when you use them merely to fill rooms. It's only when these houses are inhabited by birds that they come to life with purpose.

This analogy mirrors the relationship between T4 and T3. T4 acts as a storage unit—a repository of sorts. Yet saturating your body with T4 doesn't usually fix you. What you often need is an ample supply of active T3. In fact, your body thrives on a 1-to-4 ratio of T3 to T4. While T4 might be beneficial for patients capable of converting it to T3, many individuals struggle to efficiently or optimally convert T4 to T3 due to nutritional deficiencies, chronic stress, medications, diseases, diet, age, hormone disruptors, fluoride, chlorine, and more.

Synthroid then launched an offensive by propagating the misconception that desiccated thyroid was inconsistently mixed, inducing fear among patients that the dosages might be inadequate or excessive. Ironically, it was eventually uncovered that Synthroid itself suffered from unreliable mixing (with the FDA removing the product from shelves several times due to this very issue),[10] but by the time the facts were known, doctors en masse had already pulled their patients off natural desiccated thyroid and put them on Synthroid.

What happened to the patients who had been managing their symptoms with NDT? Well, the result was quite clear! It's highly likely that all the negative symptoms they had been effectively controlling returned. Figuratively speaking, tens of thousands of meticulously built birdhouses were shaken off their perches and returned to attics throughout the nation. Thousands of individuals found themselves grappling with fatigue, cold extremities, mental fog, persistent weight gain, and a host of other hypothyroidism symptoms. The vibrant symphony of life grew silent, and the gloomy veil of depression descended once again.

One might assume that the fact patients' symptoms returned immediately upon switching from natural thyroid to synthetic versions would have been enough to sway public opinion in favor of what genuinely works. You'd think so, but the medical community, endocrinologists, and pharmaceutical companies clung to the belief that synthetic options were the only way to go. This remains the conventional preference. However, a growing number of doctors are now turning to natural desiccated thyroid as an effective approach to treating hypothyroid patients.

SYNTHETIC ANSWERS ARE NOT WORKING

Following years of relying on synthetic T4 thyroid medication, patients are often told that their ongoing symptoms are just par for the course, as if there's no feasible solution to address them. The singular focus on T4 in the treatment of thyroid problems often results in the persistence of numerous symptoms, including aching bones, muscles, and joints; cold hands and feet; constipation; dry hair and skin; exhaustion; heavy periods; high cholesterol; lack of energy; lack of sex drive; and weight gain.

One primary reason the T4-only approach does not work well is because excessive T4 usually causes your body to make reverse T3 (rT3) from the active T3 hormones in an effort to get rid of the extra T4.[11] This means your body disposes of surplus T4 by squandering your valuable and functional T3. Comparatively, using the birdhouse analogy, rT3 seals the birdhouse shut. When that happens, the only option is to discard it. An upside of rT3 is that it frees up space for more, yet the downside is that the discarded birdhouses can never fulfill their intended purpose.

An excess of T4 typically leads to an eventual increase in rT3 levels. However, your body requires a free T3 to rT3 ratio of about 20-to-1 or even higher. When this ratio drops below that threshold, negative symptoms emerge. Allowing an imbalance of free T3 to rT3 to persist, where the ratio is less than 20-to-1, often paves the way for chronic ailments. This includes conditions such as fibromyalgia, chronic fatigue, obesity, type 2 diabetes, chronic pain syndromes, and more. Over time, chronic illnesses can exacerbate the existing imbalance.

Elevated rT3 levels should not be taken lightly, yet the TSH test might still yield a "normal range" result. This underscores the importance of testing for both rT3 and free T3. By knowing the levels of both, you can calculate your ratio.

THE THYROID HEALTH ZONE

The hormone health zone for your thyroid is well-defined. The goals are as follows:

- maximize T4-to-T3 conversion
- lower rT3 to maintain a 20-to-1 ratio of free T3 to rT3 or higher

When this happens, the typical symptoms of hypothyroidism tend to stop, reverse, or gradually fade away. When you optimize your thyroid levels, all these pieces come together. You have sufficient T4-to-T3 conversion, the ratio of T3 to rT3 is 20-to-1 or higher, and you have plenty of active T3 at work in your body.

If you're experiencing thyroid-related symptoms that persist, it usually signifies that your thyroid has not been fully optimized on one level or another. It really is as simple as that.

Maximizing T4 to T3 for more active T3

I put my patients who need to increase their free T3 levels (by maximizing the T4-to-T3 conversion process) on natural desiccated thyroid. I then check their free T3 levels within two to four weeks. If the levels improve, they often feel better, feel warmer, look more vibrant, and are happier. We proceed cautiously, adhering to the principle of "start low and go slow."

To closely monitor their progress, I advise patients to check their pulse rate daily and their axillary (armpit) temperatures in the mornings and evenings. If their pulse rate exceeds 100, I typically decrease the thyroid dose and continue monitoring their free T3. For patients sixty-five and older, as well as those with heart disease, a gentle and gradual approach is necessary to avoid stressing the heart.

I rarely prescribe a dose of natural dessicated thyroid above 30 milligrams each morning for patients eighty and older. I will occasionally prescribe NDT 30 milligrams in the morning and at noon. I recall a ninety-year-old patient with a free T3 of 1.2 and a normal TSH. After gradually adjusting her thyroid dose, her free T3 increased to 2.2. Further increases elevated her pulse to 120, prompting me to adjust the dose downward, and she did great.

If symptoms don't significantly improve after a few weeks or months, we check rT3 levels. It's possible that rT3 is blocking the T4-to-T3 conversion process.

Elevating active free T3 levels is a relatively simple yet remarkably effective procedure. Given the active role of free T3 and its significance for overall health, you usually notice when levels rise. For more information about maximizing your T4-to-T3 conversion, please read *Dr. Colbert's Hormone Health Zone.*

Lowering rT3

To effectively reduce your body's rT3 levels, it's recommended to only take liothyronine thyroid in the T3 form. Since there's already an excess of T4, there's no need for additional T4. By opting for T3 only, you naturally start lowering T4 levels, subsequently reducing rT3 levels as well. (To find a physician who is knowledgeable in this area, refer to appendix B.)

I suggest beginning with 5 micrograms of T3 (liothyronine) twice a day. If you're sensitive, you may need to start with 2.5 micrograms. Slowly increase the dosage every three to four days until you reach 25 micrograms twice a day. Maintain this dose for approximately three months. Throughout this process, monitor your pulse two to three times daily. Ensure that your resting pulse doesn't go over 100 and that you have no palpitations or irregular heartbeats. Should any of these issues arise, adjust your dose accordingly. It's essential to remain under the care of a physician well-versed in using this approach to reduce rT3.

In conjunction with this method, consider taking a multivitamin and supplementing with selenium (100–200 milligrams once per day). Following the Mediterranean-keto diet is also recommended.

Your Optimized Thyroid Levels

The recommended tests and the normal ranges are as follows:

> free T3: 2.0–4.4 pg/mL
>
> free T4: 0.8–1.8 ng/dL (optional)
>
> TSH: 0.45–4.5 µIU/L
>
> rT3: less than 15 ng/dL
>
> antibodies—TPOAbs or TgAbs: 10–20 IU/mL

When your thyroid levels are optimized, your numbers will be closer to these:

> free T3: 3.0–4.2 pg/mL
>
> free T4: 1.2–1.8 ng/dL (optional)
>
> TSH: 0.1–2.0 µIU/L or lower
>
> rT3: less than 15 ng/dL (based on the 20-to-1 ratio) antibodies—TPOAbs or TgAbs: less than 10 IU/mL free T3-to-rT3 ratio: 20-to-1 or higher

In my view, the most important numbers to know, track, and manage with your thyroid are your free T3, rT3, and TPO levels. Consequently, it is of utmost importance to undergo testing for free T3 and rT3. It's worth noting that many doctors omit these tests, so it's essential to explicitly ask for them.

Hypothyroidism or suboptimal thyroid levels affect many of us, which means you can probably identify with several of the symptoms outlined in this chapter. The encouraging news is that there's a remedy for this. You need not let these symptoms define you or dictate your life.

CHAPTER 12

FOLLOW THE ADRENALINE TRAIL

NOT EVERYONE HAS heard of the adrenal glands, but everyone has heard about adrenaline. This hormone, known for triggering the fight-or-flight response, goes by the name of epinephrine as well. It gives your body and muscles a boost, facilitating extra blood flow, increased heart rate, pupil dilation, and the release of blood sugar. This redirection of resources steers the blood away from the skin and digestive system, channeling it toward the muscles and brain.

Situated just above your kidneys, the adrenal glands aren't solely responsible for producing adrenaline; they also manufacture cortisol along with other hormones, playing a major role in your endocrine system.

Cortisol is generated to aid the body's reaction to stress. Small increases in cortisol will usually give you a burst of energy, improve memory and immunity, and even lower your sensitivity to pain. While adrenaline might jumpstart your system's response to stress, cortisol is needed to help your body respond to stress in a healthy way.

Sustaining a heightened state of stress is not good for your health. The persistent, prolonged release of excessive cortisol in response to everyday stresses can harm our bodies over time.

Even a mild overproduction of cortisol leaves symptoms behind. This "adrenaline trail" is leading millions of people off a health-ruining cliff!

THE ROLE OF ADRENALS IN YOUR HEALTH

When it comes to your adrenals, hormones, and overall health, I have come to this conclusion: you will never balance—much less optimize—your other hormones until you balance your adrenal hormones. Quite simply, your hormone health requires healthy adrenals. That is because poor adrenal function can make your hormone issues worse and delay any forward progress you might be making. While at times the adrenals are the underlying issue, more often they act like gas or accelerant to an already burning fire. They usually make things worse, and putting a fire out with gas is not a good strategy.

Regrettably, many doctors do not typically test adrenal function, which could explain why so many adrenal issues go undetected. When the approach is to only address a problem once it reaches a certain level of severity, an adrenal test is of little value. However, when the focus shifts from masking and temporary solutions to repairing and preventing the problem, getting your adrenals checked might offer some insight into your symptoms and possible hormone issues.

As I said, the adrenals supply you with adrenaline and cortisol to aid your body in coping with stress. Yet prolonged exposure to cortisol negatively impacts your body, and this connects with my previous discussion on thyroid hormones, as well as what we will discuss in forthcoming chapters. Allow me to explain.

1. Excessive cortisol blocks T4-to-T3 conversion. Yes, you read that correctly. The vital conversion process that gives your body its much-needed active T3 thyroid hormone is slowed down sometimes significantly by the extra cortisol in your system. You could literally be hypothyroid, with the many unpleasant symptoms that go with it, all because your adrenals are producing too much cortisol.

2. Excessive cortisol increases rT3 production. Increasing the production of rT3 in your body wrecks the necessary 20-to-1 ratio of free T3 to rT3, and that in turn usually results in a very sick thyroid. Some nasty hypothyroid symptoms and chronic diseases are right behind it. Of course, that in turn only makes things worse.

3. Excessive cortisol lowers testosterone. This also is big news! In the following chapters I will discuss the importance of testosterone for both men and women, but for now, suffice it to say that you absolutely do not want to

lower testosterone levels. The symptoms of low testosterone are some of the worst.

4. Excessive cortisol increases conversion of testosterone into estrogen. Men certainly don't want more estrogen in their bodies, but neither do women want this type of estrogen elevated. The type of estrogen created is usually estrone, which is the so-called "old lady estrogen" that usually causes more belly fat and weight gain. The testosterone-to-estrogen balance is vital for both men and women, but cortisol ruins it. I will discuss more about estrogen for men and women in later chapters.

———

Because most hormones operate in a feedback loop, a decrease in your hormone levels typically triggers an increase in cortisol production, and the more cortisol your body pumps out, the more it messes up your other hormones. This vicious cycle never ends, but your adrenals cannot keep it up forever. The relentless overproduction of cortisol eventually wears out the adrenal glands, leading to adrenal fatigue and burnout. Cortisol levels generally plummet in this scenario, which increases your risk of inflammatory and autoimmune disease, essentially inviting them into your body.

The negative impact of blocked conversion of T4 to T3, increased production of reverse T3 (rT3), lowered testosterone levels, and the transformation of testosterone into estrogen create an array of undesirable symptoms. Unfortunately, doctors frequently encounter these symptoms in their practice, often diagnosing them as obesity, dementia, osteoporosis, sarcopenia, hypertension, depression, fibromyalgia, or type 2 diabetes. Sadly, they frequently overlook the underlying cause—adrenal burnout or adrenal fatigue.

As if that's not enough, when your adrenals are fatigued, they produce less of the anti-aging hormone dehydroepiandrosterone (DHEA). This hormone, also synthesized in the adrenal glands, plays a crucial role in promoting muscle development and keeping you looking and feeling young.

The problem for all of us is that after age twenty, our DHEA levels drop by about 2 percent each year.[1] But if you speed up the DHEA decline by adding adrenal fatigue, you get lower DHEA hormone levels sooner than normal.

As you can see, your adrenals play a pivotal role in your overall health. If your adrenal glands are hurting, so are you.

WHAT CAUSES ADRENAL FATIGUE?

You may be thinking, "I'm not an adrenaline junkie, and I don't have daily scary situations that get my adrenaline pumping. So why would my adrenals even have an issue?"

I admit that heart-pounding, adrenaline-charged moments are few and far between, and that's certainly for the best. Nevertheless, your body has other strains, stressors, and concerns that never give your stress-response system a break. Cortisol is naturally released to restore calm during short-term, high-alert scenarios. However, when there is no end to the loop or stress, the cortisol keeps flowing. It's like your alarm button is stuck in the "on" position, and cortisol levels get higher and higher.

High cortisol can disturb crucial bodily functions and pave the way for problems such as elevated blood sugar, high blood pressure, decreased thyroid function, and adrenal fatigue.

Stress is an inevitable part of all our lives. Total avoidance is impossible, signifying that each of us is placing a strain on our adrenal glands. It's imperative that we take time to recharge and rejuvenate our adrenals, lest we develop a host of symptoms and diseases to deal with down the road. Astonishingly, I've even come across cases of teenagers suffering from adrenal burnout. That's not the ideal path to be headed down. That is also why my medical experience has led me to believe this cortisol loop pertains to us all.

TEST YOUR ADRENAL HEALTH

There are several ways to screen your adrenal function, and you might consider conducting more than one test. I've discovered the following three tests to be very accurate, easy, and noninvasive.

Adrenal test 1: seven-day temperature test

This test can be conducted in the comfort of your own home, and it serves as a valuable means to assess both your thyroid and adrenal health. Measure your temperature every three hours, starting when you wake up. If you've eaten or engaged in physical activity at the three-hour mark, allow thirty minutes to pass before taking your temperature. The objective is to identify any fluctuations in your temperature readings.

If your daily body temperature average is 98.6°F, which is normal, but if you fluctuated 0.2–0.3° between measurements, then your adrenals probably have an issue but not your thyroid. However, if your temperature is below normal but steady, then it's more likely a thyroid issue, and your adrenals may be fine. All combined (low temperature with fluctuations) means you most likely have both adrenal and thyroid issues.

Adrenal test 2: saliva test

Cortisol levels exhibit variations throughout the day, so the saliva test collects your saliva four to six times in a day, then gives you an average cortisol score. Basically, you spit into a plastic vial at four-hour intervals. Similar to the seven-day temperature test, wait thirty minutes after food or exercise before collecting the sample. Then send the vial through the mail to the medical service provider.

I believe this is more accurate than a blood test for two reasons: (1) a blood test only measures your cortisol levels once, and they could simply be high or low at that moment, and (2) the needle prick from a blood test causes enough stress to affect cortisol levels, but there is no stress in a saliva test. (See appendix B for more information about the saliva test.)

Adrenal test 3: blood pressure screening test

The blood pressure test is usually done in a doctor's office. While lying down, check your blood pressure. Then check it while you are standing. Normally your systolic blood pressure should increase 8–10 points when standing. If your blood pressure drops by 10 points or more, you probably have low adrenal function. Usually the greater the drop, the lower the adrenal function.

Because there are many recommended tests for adrenals, you will have to choose the one you prefer. I usually recommend the blood pressure screen and the saliva test because it only takes one day to complete both. At the mention of adrenal testing, most doctors will recommend the adrenocorticotropic hormone (ACTH) stimulation test or more tests, such as a blood serum/cortisol test or a twenty-four-hour urine collection test for cortisol. Unfortunately, these don't give the best results for showing adrenal fatigue.

SLEEP APNEA AND ADRENALS

It is not just a nuisance. If you suffer from sleep apnea, your brain is likely starved for oxygen, and you have unknowingly signed up for almost every disease. Take a moment to answer:

Do you snore at night? Y/N

Do you stop breathing at night? Y/N

Do you wake up gasping for air? Y/N

Do you have a dry mouth in the morning? Y/N

Do you wake up in the morning exhausted? Y/N

People with sleep apnea are usually bone-tired, have no energy, and cannot seem to get recharged. That is adrenal fatigue in action. They also have a higher risk for high blood pressure, memory loss, atrial fibrillation, diabetes, cancer, heart issues, dementia, and more, all because of the lack of oxygen. If you have sleep apnea, you cannot make it into the hormone health zone. You are stuck. You must break free of sleep apnea first.

Step 1 is to get a sleep study such as the SNAP Diagnostics sleep study in the comfort of your home.

Step 2 is to get more oxygen with a CPAP (or BiPAP) machine. Armed with sufficient oxygen, the adrenals do not have to work as hard, blood pressure comes down, and losing weight is easier.

Step 3 is to use diet (e.g., the healthy keto diet) and moderate exercise to assist the healing process.

Step 4 is to optimize hormone levels. Many patients eventually do away with their CPAP machines entirely at that point.

TREATMENT PLAN FOR ADRENAL HEALTH

An important detail few know is that our stress-response system is basically like a timer. After the adrenaline boost, it takes about ninety minutes for it to reset. If you reset it (e.g., fight or flight, address the issue, choose to forgive, reframe it, move on, walk in peace, and so on), then the timer turns off. If you don't stop it, the timer will keep ticking, and cortisol levels may stay elevated. This can go on for years until your adrenals crash and you develop adrenal fatigue with low cortisol levels.

Whenever you choose to remain too busy, multitasking, moving too fast, offended, angry, depressed, and so on, you allow the timer to keep running. You must learn how to stop the timer and then learn how to treat your adrenals. In addition to the mental and emotional side of adrenal health, there is the practical treatment side as well, which includes the following:

Sleep and rest

Get a good night's sleep: seven to nine hours and sometimes ten hours each night for those with severe adrenal fatigue. Learn to rest. Find things you enjoy doing that make you feel recharged. Overcome insomnia with natural supplements such as melatonin, L-theanine, magnesium threonate, or micronized progesterone for women. (See appendix B.)

Diet

The Mediterranean-keto diet is ideal. Drink about 1–1½ quarts of alkaline water per day and avoid excessive caffeine.

Nutrition

Include vitamin supplements (B_5, C, and D), selenium, iodine, iron for women, zinc, magnesium, and B complex. Adaptogens or adaptogenic herbs can balance (increase or decrease) cortisol levels, based on your body's needs, and that is healthy. Some natural adaptogenic herbs include ginseng (American, Asian, or Siberian), rhodiola, ashwagandha, licorice, rhaponticum, reishi, and many more.

Adrenal glandular extracts from pigs, sheep, or cows are adrenal rebuilders in pill form and may be taken one to three times a day. You can usually get them in most health food stores or online. Standard Process has two very good adrenal rebuilders: (1) Drenamin and (2) Adrenal Desiccated. The dose is usually two or three tablets in the morning and two or three tablets at noon. Nutri-West also has a good adrenal rebuilder for men called DSF Formula (destress formula).

Another option is a Myers' cocktail IV, which contains vitamins and minerals that help support and reboot the adrenals. It's usually given once a week, and many of my patients have restored their adrenals with Myers' IVs. Optimizing testosterone levels also helps to reboot the adrenal glands.

Exercise

Find an exercise program you enjoy, one that does not burn all the little energy you have left. If you are suffering from severe adrenal fatigue, very mild exercises are recommended, such as stretching and leisurely walks as able (not necessarily daily) for only ten to thirty minutes. If exercise leaves you exhausted, decrease your time and intensity of exercise. You should feel refreshed after exercising and not exhausted. Some patients with severe adrenal fatigue need to wait a few months before exercising to help recharge their adrenals.

Some patients have adrenal issues and no thyroid problems at all. All they usually need is a good multivitamin with adequate B vitamins, especially B_5, and maybe some rhodiola (an adaptogen) and to follow the above treatment plan for adrenal health.

For individuals dealing with adrenal fatigue, these practical components often prove sufficient to reinvigorate their adrenals. While the journey to restoring normal adrenal function will typically take a few months to a year, it's a process well worth the new habit formation.

However, when people have pushed their adrenal fatigue to the level of adrenal exhaustion, they will usually need additional help to reboot their adrenal glands. This also happens to people who are chronically ill (with fibromyalgia, Lyme disease, cancer, and so on), as the severity of their illness drains their adrenals.

Regardless of the root cause, severe adrenal exhaustion frequently calls for hydrocortisone (cortisol) therapy. This entails consuming minor doses of hydrocortisone throughout the day, following a pattern that mirrors your body's natural cortisol production rhythm. It's crucial to obtain a prescription for hydrocortisone. In my approach, I first check a salivary adrenal panel, which is the best test to measure cortisol. Like the slow trickle charge for batteries, hydrocortisone slowly recharges the adrenals over a period of several months. To avoid GI upset, take hydrocortisone with a small amount of food.

The good news about your adrenal health is that once you restore adrenal function, you can eventually discontinue hydrocortisone medication. For most people, several months of taking 2.5–5 milligrams of hydrocortisone medication during meals, with an additional 10 milligrams during breakfast, is usually enough to reset their system. (I steer clear of prescribing prednisone, a synthetic glucocorticoid that is four to five times more potent than hydrocortisone and lasts a lot longer, usually twelve hours or more, because long-term use is associated with a multitude of side effects. Bioidentical hydrocortisone provides physiological doses of cortisol, which is the amount your body is supposed to make.)

These are relatively small dosages, yet they work well to restore energy levels, boost immune function, decrease inflammation, and restore the adrenals. All in all, hydrocortisone helps restore the adrenals. My typical regimen is to start patients with 10 milligrams at around 8:00 a.m. with food, followed by 5 milligrams at noon, another 2.5–5 milligrams at 4:00 p.m., and rarely 2.5–5 milligrams at bedtime. Many of these patients also benefit from weekly Myers' IVs.

The prospect of using medication for a short time and then discontinuing it has considerable appeal for most patients. This certainly applies to rebooting the adrenal glands. By contrast, individuals with adrenal issues who begin antianxiety medications often find themselves taking those drugs indefinitely!

THE HORMONE HEALTH ZONE FOR ADRENAL HEALTH

Stress wreaks havoc on our bodies, particularly on our adrenal glands. If stressors aren't managed effectively, they gradually manifest as symptoms. It's hard to believe, but 75–90 percent of doctor visits stem from stress-related issues.[2] As we age, our hormone levels typically decline, often reaching borderline low or low levels, further compounding the impact of stress.

One very encouraging factor in your adrenal health is that when you optimize your hormone levels, especially testosterone with hormone pellet therapy, it is usually enough to reboot your adrenal glands as well! The optimal hormone health zone for your adrenals is connected directly to your thyroid and testosterone hormone levels. Given that cortisol from the adrenals persistently chips away at your thyroid and testosterone, recharging your adrenals is a huge boost to your testosterone and thyroid levels. In essence, by positively influencing one, you're positively impacting all three hormones simultaneously.

Caution: if your physician prescribes an excessive dose of thyroid hormone, it can also deplete your adrenal glands. That's why I keep the free T3 in the range of 3.0–4.2 pg/mL.

Believe me, the results of optimizing testosterone and thyroid function while rebooting your adrenals are often remarkable. Most of the negative symptoms we've discussed so far are directly influenced by these three. So when you optimize these three types of hormones (testosterone, thyroid, adrenal), you are potentially fixing the list of symptoms along with them.

When it comes to optimizing your hormone levels and healing your adrenals, let me share two secrets. First, for many men and women, optimizing testosterone levels often leads to improvement or resolution of adrenal issues, frequently without the need for hydrocortisone. Second, for women, taking bioidentical micronized progesterone at night usually helps them sleep like a baby. It also helps them grow beautiful hair, reduces irritability, gives a deep sense of calm, and is the answer to managing PMS symptoms. Clearly, optimizing hormone levels yields benefits across the spectrum, particularly if rejuvenating your adrenals is a part of the equation.

CHAPTER 13

THE THREE HORMONE DOMINOES IN WOMEN

FOR MOST WOMEN, a decrease in three key hormones usually begins around age forty. The process might be gradual, but it is relentless. The decline can be accelerated by stress, medications, chronic illness, endocrine disruptors, menopause, or removal of the ovaries. *Testosterone*, *progesterone*, and *estradiol* are like three hormone dominoes. Once they begin to fall, no diet or weight loss program, no pill or drink will get your curves back, reverse wrinkling, wash away the cellulite, or control the host of other negative symptoms.

It's called "aging" by most people, including many doctors, and women are told to accept the sagging features, the expanding waistlines, and less muscle tone because "that's what happens when you get older." Even the irritability, lack of libido, and depression are included in the package and are usually treated with medication, especially antidepressants. But this doesn't have to be the case. To explain why, let's start by looking at each domino a little more closely.

Domino 1: testosterone

Testosterone is usually the first domino to fall. Though essential for women's hormone balance, around age thirty-five to forty it usually starts to decline rapidly. (At age forty, women usually have half the testosterone they had at twenty.) It is part of a woman's natural shift from a reproductive to a nonreproductive stage of life, but still, it's no fun!

Domino 2: progesterone

Then five to ten years later, at approximately age forty-five, progesterone levels begin to lower as women hit menopause and their ovaries hit or miss with progesterone production. When progesterone starts to decline, a host of ailments come right with it, including bloating, breast tenderness, fatigue, heavy bleeding, joint pain, moodiness, PMS, poor sleep, hair loss, and water retention. As the progesterone peters out, the only hormone left is estrogen.

Domino 3: estrogen (estradiol)

At this point, approximately five years later (typically between ages fifty and fifty-five), testosterone is usually so low that it has virtually no impact on the woman's body. If stress and medications are also in the system (e.g., antidepressants, cholesterol-lowering drugs, antianxiety drugs, insomnia drugs, and so on), then you can forget about testosterone. It's usually gone.

With progesterone also on a steep decline, there is one hormone left that seeks to rule the woman's body: estrogen. That might not sound very bad, since estrogen is known as the female hormone, but there are three main types of estrogen: E1 (estrone), E2 (estradiol), and E3 (estriol), and it's not the good type of estrogen that wins the battle. Estrone is the "old lady estrogen," or as I prefer to call it, the "elderly estrogen," and is the main estrogen in the female after menopause. It characteristically causes muscle to be replaced with fat (especially in the belly and back), raises bad cholesterol, increases the risk for breast cancer and heart disease, and contributes to sagging and painful breasts, sagging skin, obesity, irritability, and poor memory. Even though the other types of estrogen are higher during childbearing years, eventually estrone will rule. It always does.

THE ANSWER TO CELLULITE

Low oxygen levels cause a pocket or dimple in the skin. The skin needs more oxygen and greater blood flow, and the answer is more testosterone. Optimized testosterone levels reduce and sometimes totally remove cellulite.

Estradiol, the pretty and youthful estrogen, the estrogen that all women want, will fight valiantly for a decade or more, but with no support from testosterone or progesterone, and constant internal attacks from stress, medications, endocrine disruptors, poor nutrition, a lack of exercise, and more, it will inevitably give way to estrone.

And estrone will rule with an iron fist! It is merciless. If you thought the loss of progesterone brought with it a wave of unpleasant symptoms, estrone dominance is far worse. Common symptoms I see every day include anxiety, belly fat, cellulite, dry vagina, hair loss, hot flashes, insomnia, fatigue, poor memory, recurrent UTIs, saggy breasts and skin, thin skin, and wrinkles.

You are no doubt wondering if there is any good news. Yes, there is! Dominoes that have fallen can be righted again. For that matter, they didn't need to fall in the first place. This means you can get your body back! You can get your health back! You can get your dreams back! I have found with optimized levels of estradiol and testosterone, you can keep your healthy-looking body into old age, and that includes all the benefits associated with it.

The negative symptoms you dislike so much can usually be reversed and many times eliminated. So the next time you hear, "Well, that's what happens as you age," you can breathe a sigh of relief because it doesn't apply to you!

TESTOSTERONE IN WOMEN

The first hormone women need to optimize is testosterone. Although women produce a lot less testosterone than men (about 10 percent of what men produce), having sufficient testosterone in our bodies is equally essential for everyone.[1] After all, testosterone "is the central hormone in the aging process."[2]

Few women are aware that their bodies contain a substantial amount of testosterone, particularly during their youthful years. Throughout their twenties and thirties, their testosterone levels remain within the normal range. However, the decline usually becomes evident after the age of forty.

Being within the normal range is certainly commendable. Yet, as we've discussed, various factors, such as aging, ovary removal, menopause, medications, and stress, can progressively lower testosterone levels. Should you find yourself positioned toward the lower end of these ranges or even below them, your body is essentially signaling a need for increased testosterone.

Regrettably, most medical practitioners are trained to prescribe only modest doses of estradiol, often in pill form (which is less than ideal), and completely omit testosterone. In fact, it's common for doctors to overlook hormone-related issues entirely. They may present you with the "normal ranges" (where you might still fall), and if you happen to have low levels, they typically prescribe medication to manage the symptoms.

However, this approach will not restore your health. What your body truly requires is bioidentical hormone therapy. It might be necessary to seek out another healthcare provider, someone willing to address your low testosterone symptoms with bioidentical testosterone.

In my experience, utilizing pellets to elevate testosterone levels has proven to be highly effective and efficient. Pellets lead to rapid increases in levels, and the convenience of not requiring another treatment for three to four months, and occasionally even six months, is notable. If pellets are not within budget, the next favorable option is testosterone injections, followed by testosterone creams. Injections are typically administered once or twice a week. Testosterone cream can be applied behind the knee daily or directly to the female genital area every other day or three times per week. In certain cases, I've also prescribed a sublingual testosterone tablet compounded at a specialized pharmacy.

Through the use of pellets, women can witness their total testosterone levels climb to approximately 70–100 ng/dL in just a week! Subsequently, maintaining testosterone levels around 70–100 ng/dL is often ideal for most women, and sometimes even higher. This results in a remarkable transformation—better health, bone growth, muscle replacing fat, improved brain function, a stronger heart, and rapidly increased energy levels.

As for free testosterone, which is the active testosterone, doctors (especially endocrinologists) will recommend very low levels according to your age, such as 0.2–5.0 pg/mL for those ages eighteen through sixty-nine and 0.3–5.0 pg/mL for women ages seventy through eighty-nine. Women whose numbers match their recommendations usually also have matching low-testosterone symptoms! The recommended normal ranges for total testosterone and free testosterone in women are as follows:

- total testosterone: 2.0–45 ng/dL
- free testosterone: 0.2–5.0 pg/mL

According to some sources, a normal testosterone level for women ages twenty to thirty is 13–71 ng/dL. When your testosterone levels are optimized (pushed to the upper ranges or a little higher) to the levels you were at when you were in your twenties, your numbers will be closer to these:

- total testosterone: 70–100 ng/dL (higher for those with osteoporosis or sarcopenia)
- free testosterone: 5–10 pg/mL

Remarkable transformations unfold at these optimized levels. In instances where my female patients contend with sarcopenia (muscle weakness) and osteoporosis, I might strive to elevate their total testosterone levels to as high as 150–200 ng/dL and sometimes higher. This elevation often helps reverse sarcopenia and osteoporosis in a significant number of them. From my perspective, testosterone replacement stands out as the superior approach to combating osteoporosis, with minimal side effects as compared to most osteoporosis medications.

I recommend women in their forties start monitoring their testosterone levels. The opportune time to begin optimizing testosterone levels is when hormone levels dip below 50–60 percent of the upper range or when symptoms start emerging, usually at age forty. Typically, when levels drop below 50 percent, persistent low-testosterone symptoms manifest. When you are attuned to your body, you can diligently track changes as they occur.

PROGESTERONE ANSWERS FOR WOMEN

It's important to remember that progesterone is the second hormone domino to topple in women. This usually occurs within a span of merely five to ten years after the rapid decline of testosterone has begun. Renowned board-certified ob-gyn specialist Dr. Gary Donovitz states that by age forty a woman's progesterone production may have decreased by 80 percent.[3] That is a massive drop! To be left with only 20 percent of what is normal is never going to be enough to meet life's demands.

Like other hormones, progesterone is shrouded by myths and apprehensions. However, just as with other hormones, more and more studies are being done to find the truth, the real value, behind progesterone. That includes everything from type (bioidentical versus synthetic) to dosage and lasting effects. Bioidentical, micronized progesterone protects women against breast cancer; however, synthetic progestin (the synthetic counterfeit for bioidentical, micronized progesterone) increases one's risk of breast cancer.

I frequently caution patients whose primary care doctors or ob-gyns prescribe synthetic progesterone: "Do not take it. You are increasing your risks for breast cancer, heart attacks, strokes, blood clots, and more. If the progesterone is not micronized and bioidentical, do not fill your prescription." That is how serious this is, but as always patients make their own choices.

Both medical practitioners and patients need to remember that hormone optimization entails returning these hormones to the upper range of normal. That should not scare anyone.

For women with a uterus, progesterone is essential, as it shields the uterus from abnormal bleeding and guards against uterine cancer, particularly when estrogen replacement therapy is in play. But what if a woman has undergone a hysterectomy or entered menopause? It's a valid question, and my response is, "Do women want to sleep better, reduce depression and irritability, have thick, beautiful hair, and minimize mood swings?" The need for progesterone doesn't disappear, regardless of the season of life a woman is in.

Women who have had difficulty conceiving or suffered miscarriages definitely need to watch their progesterone levels. Progesterone helps them become and stay pregnant, while also protecting the uterus during pregnancy. When women voice concerns about infertility, I not only check their progesterone levels but also their thyroid function. An underactive thyroid is a sure way to keep a woman from conceiving. I also check for an MTHFR gene mutation.

When women have too little progesterone, they often have too much estrogen and are usually estrogen dominant. This typically results in emotional upheaval, irritability, anxiety, and restlessness. This is particularly prevalent around the age of forty-five when the second hormone domino (progesterone) falls. When progesterone levels are optimized (alongside estrogen, thyroid, and testosterone levels, as the goal is to optimize all hormones simultaneously), the body is usually calmer and not ruled by the emotional side of the often-dominating estrogen hormone.

Among the most frequent symptoms in women with low progesterone are irritability, poor sleep quality, and PMS. Whether or not they have had a hysterectomy, optimizing progesterone levels typically brings relief from these symptoms. This isn't about merely "patching" things up; it's about genuine resolution. With properly optimized progesterone levels, I've observed that these symptoms seldom resurface, much to the delight of women seeking relief.

THE PROGESTERONE HEALTH ZONE FOR WOMEN

According to LabCorp, the ranges for women's progesterone hormone levels fluctuate a lot. Consider these numbers:[4]

- follicular phase: 0.1–0.9 ng/mL
- luteal phase: 1.8–23.9 ng/mL
- ovulatory phase: 0.1–12.0 ng/mL

And if pregnant, those numbers change even more:

- first trimester: 11.0–44.3 ng/mL
- second trimester: 25.4–83.3 ng/mL
- third trimester: 58.7–214.0 ng/mL

And if postmenopausal:

- 0.0–0.1 ng/mL

If you are postmenopausal or have undergone a hysterectomy, the goal is to replicate the hormone levels you had in your twenties. During that period, the normal upper range was between 10–20 ng/mL, and that is the range we strive to achieve once more.

The recommended "normal" ranges for progesterone in women are as follows:

- progesterone as adult: 0.1–25 ng/mL
- progesterone when pregnant: 10–290 ng/mL
- progesterone when postmenopausal: 0.1–1.0 ng/mL

For pregnant women, keeping progesterone levels high enough to maintain the pregnancy is the goal. The optimized progesterone levels for premenopausal and postmenopausal women should be closer to these:

- progesterone as an adult: 5–20 ng/mL
- progesterone when postmenopausal: 5–20 ng/mL

Most women who need progesterone therapy usually fall in the post-menopausal category, so returning their progesterone levels to 5–20 ng/mL is exactly what the body needs. Micronized progesterone may cause some women to gain belly fat if the dose is 125 milligrams or higher.

How is it applied—with pills, sublingual tabs, or creams? For bioidentical progesterone, one of the best methods is with sublingual tabs under the tongue before bedtime. The sublingual tabs or troches are easy to use, inexpensive, very effective, and come in varying dosages.

The same method works for women who are trying to get pregnant. Approximate sublingual or oral dosages are as follows:

- raising progesterone hormone levels toward optimization: 75–200 milligrams at bedtime (I start women over sixty-five at lower dosages such as 75–100 milligrams and monitor progesterone levels.)

- raising progesterone hormone levels to aid in getting pregnant: 50–75 milligrams daily (days twelve to twenty-six of menstrual cycle)

Using sublingual bioidentical progesterone tabs before bedtime often induces sleepiness. This effect can be particularly beneficial if you're a woman dealing with depression or a chronic illness. A good night's sleep is vital.

Micronized progesterone is created from plants and matches the progesterone naturally present in a woman's body. As expected, synthetic progesterone does not and causes many of the adverse side effects already mentioned. Bioidentical progesterone therapy is one of the most powerful health tools available. That means enduring a life of misery is no longer the only option.

ESTROGEN ANSWERS FOR WOMEN

Women often feel as if estrogen has unexpectedly turned against them. Their "young lady" feminine features from one estrogen (estradiol) suddenly in a few short years turned into "elderly lady," not-so-flattering features from another estrogen (estrone). What's really going on?

The puzzle starts to unravel when we acknowledge the presence of three distinct types of estrogen operating within your body. Women also need to grasp the impact of menopause—simply put, it shuts down the ovaries. They stop releasing eggs and stop optimal production of hormones.

Once women transition into menopause, the ovaries suddenly stop producing estradiol. That means very little estrone is converted to estradiol. (If your ovaries have been removed, you have almost a complete and sudden stop of estrone-to-estradiol conversion!) While other parts of the body, such as the liver, adrenals, and fatty tissue, continue to generate estrone, there is a notable absence of substantial estrone-to-estradiol conversion across the body. This phenomenon paves the way for the emergence of undesirable symptoms.

In essence, here's the situation: after menopause, the youthful estrogen you desire most (estradiol) essentially ceases production. While trace amounts of estradiol might still undergo conversion in certain body areas, it never reaches the same levels as before menopause.

However, the good news is that you can restore your body to its optimal 2-to-1 ratio. You start reversing the aging process. And the solution might pleasantly surprise you.

THE ESTROGEN HEALTH ZONE FOR WOMEN

Optimizing your estrogen hormone levels focuses not on boosting your estradiol (E2) levels to the 2-to-1 ratio over estrone (E1) but on lowering your follicle-stimulating hormone (FSH) levels to 23 IU/L (international units per liter) and for some to 50 IU/L or less. Let me explain.

Estradiol can be a double-edged sword for some women. High normal levels of estradiol can trigger dysfunctional uterine bleeding, intense and painful menstruation, severe menstrual cramps, fibrocystic breast disease, and the resurgence of periods in postmenopausal women. Furthermore, it serves as the driving force behind numerous gynecological issues, including uterine fibroids, endometriosis, and certain female cancers. Due to these considerations, I opt not to optimize estrogen levels in women, and some women may even need to abstain from estrogens, particularly those with a history of breast, ovarian, or uterine cancer. Women with endometriosis and fibroids require much smaller amounts of estradiol so that it doesn't reactivate their disease.

I can usually help women avoid most or all the above symptoms by focusing on the FSH, which is a pituitary hormone. When a woman's FSH level is greater than 23 IU/L on two separate blood tests two weeks apart, then they are menopausal and no longer fertile. They can usually stop birth control pills without fear of getting pregnant. After menopause, my goal is to give enough estradiol to suppress the FSH level to 23 IU/L or less. I find that estradiol pellets usually work the best at getting FSH levels to 23 or less but for some to 50 or less.

When the FSH is less than 23, usually almost all the main symptoms of menopause are resolved, including vaginal dryness, hot flashes, night sweats, painful intercourse, poor sleep, and mood disturbances. Hot flashes and night sweats are usually caused by a surge of FSH, which triggers the sympathetic nervous system to release adrenaline, which in turn causes the stress response to be stimulated with an increased heart rate.

There is another aspect of the estrogen optimization process that you must consider. As women transition into menopause and the interplay between estrone and estradiol begins, something happens behind the scenes that often goes unnoticed. Two pituitary hormones essential for reproduction, follicle-stimulating hormone (FSH) and luteinizing hormone (LH), begin to increase with no opposition. The less estradiol in your system, the higher these two (especially LH) will climb. Usually the higher these hormone levels climb, the more pronounced the potential for brain degeneration.[5]

Did you catch that? Keeping these two hormones in check by optimizing your hormone levels, especially estradiol and testosterone, could help prevent Alzheimer's and dementia.[6] Who needs another reason to optimize hormone levels?

With all the known benefits of optimizing estradiol levels, spanning from metabolism and weight loss to heart health and disease prevention, I find it surprising that most doctors stop all forms of estrogen therapy just ten years after menopause. This practice might stem from the notion that after prolonged usage, the risks could outweigh the benefits. Nonetheless, in the case of bioidentical estrogen, I've observed that this isn't necessarily true. (Moreover, if physicians do prescribe estrogen, it's often the pregnant horse hormone Premarin derived from pregnant mares' urine, which the body struggles to utilize effectively, resulting in numerous adverse effects.)

Consequently, countless women around the age of sixty undergo an abrupt and involuntary acceleration of aging along with cognitive decline. The truth is this rapid aging and the associated adverse symptoms need not occur. By optimizing hormone levels, women can usually stop the clock and even turn back time!

For estrogen, there are several application options depending on your needs. Before I explain each application, I want to mention that in addition to taking estrogen, women (like men) need to take DIM, a natural supplement made from broccoli, to decrease estrone and help restore the 2-to-1 estradiol-to-estrone ratio. A 150 milligram tablet once or twice each day (twice a day for men) is sufficient. (See appendix B.)

Creams

Creams provide a swift, convenient, and typically cost-effective solution. Generally, a single application per day suffices. For instance, you can apply an estriol wrinkle cream once daily. First moisten your hands with water, and then apply 1 mL of the cream to your face, neck, and the backs of your hands. Estriol tends to work marvels in conjunction with collagen. And after a couple of months, there is often a huge difference. Some patients tell me their friends believed they had a face-lift. A compounding pharmacy makes it for my patients, and we playfully call it wrinkle cream.

Typically, creams require just one application per day. Nevertheless, as women age their skin's capacity to absorb estrogen may decline. Consequently, over time adjustments might be needed, such as increasing the dosage or altering the application method.

Another cream is made to address vaginal dryness and atrophy. Women with this condition are miserable, but the estradiol cream works wonders in restoring the woman's vaginal fluids. Creams can be applied to the labia and vagina or may be applied to the skin. I usually recommend an estradiol/estriol cream in a 1-to-1 ratio (such as Biest) two or three times a week, and for some, daily. Some women can only tolerate the estriol cream (they are less likely to start their periods again or have cramps, spotting, or breast tenderness, potential side effects of estradiol), which is the weakest estrogen, and is applied to the labia and vagina only two or three times a week.

Estradiol Patches

Estradiol patches also are easy, quick, and usually inexpensive. These adhesive patches remain effective for several days, meaning you may only need one or two per week. However, some women report that the patches may come off following showering or swimming, while others may experience itching. The experience can vary depending on the individual.

Sublingual tabs

Sublingual tablets offer another swift, convenient, and typically cost-effective alternative. A tablet once a day under the tongue or, for enhanced absorption, between the lower lip and gum, dissolves within minutes, making this approach efficient, easy, and problem-free.

If your FSH level remains above 23 despite optimizing doses through the methods mentioned previously, then pellets are the best option available.

Shots

Once-a-week estradiol shots are quick and easy, usually not painful at all when using tiny needles, and inexpensive. I rarely recommend them because pellets are superior in my opinion.

Pellets

Pellets, inserted under the skin within a matter of minutes, prove to be virtually painless and maintain their efficacy for a span of three to five months. This approach offers the most effective delivery of both estrogen and testosterone, ensuring a consistent dosage release. Although it comes with a higher price tag compared to other methods, it boasts exceptional effectiveness and often leads to a swifter and more consistent reduction in FSH levels than any alternative.

Again, the method of application is up to you. Talk with your doctor. Depending on the steps you need to take to optimize your estrogen levels, you can use one application method or another. Once you have chosen your preferred method of application, bioidentical hormones will do wonders in your body, usually bringing such dramatic change that women feel youthful and feminine again.

Whatever your age, it is never too late to start. But if I were to outline a proposed schedule for women, it would look something like this:

- At age forty, or perhaps sooner, optimize testosterone levels.
- At age forty-five start on progesterone.
- At age fifty (the average age for menopause) start on estrogen.

And you can keep this up until you are 100 or 120. Basically, bioidentical hormone replacement therapy can keep you young and healthy for as long as you want. For women who have had breast cancer and can no longer use estrogen or progesterone, I use testosterone pellets that contain the estrogen blocker Anastrozole. These pellets protect them from recurrence of breast cancer and help to restore their energy, vitality, and libido.

WHEN ESTRADIOL IS RESTORED TO POWER

Once your body is reestablished at its desired 2-to-1 ratio of estradiol to estrone, with FSH levels dropping to 23 IU/L or below, a revitalization often occurs. Numerous women describe this phenomenon as if a switch has been flipped, and their bodies come alive. While your symptoms may vary, optimizing hormone levels typically leads to an improvement across the board. However, keep in mind that each individual's body responds uniquely, and outcomes can differ from one person to the next—this is consistently the case.

CHAPTER 14

WHAT MEN NEED TO KNOW

IT MIGHT COME as a surprise, but men also require estrogen. Achieving the right balance is crucial, as estrogen is beneficial in the right amounts but can be detrimental if you have too much or too little. The proper amount of estradiol is good for bone strength, sperm count, cholesterol metabolism, a healthy libido, and clear cognitive function in the brain, among other recognized benefits for men.

However, a surplus of estrogen is often more common in men over fifty. This occurs when testosterone levels drop due to factors such as aging, obesity, sedentary lifestyles, lack of exercise, stress, exposure to endocrine disruptors, and more. Excess estrogen has been found to promote abnormal blood clot formation. Elevated estrogen levels also may increase the risk of stroke.

As testosterone decreases, estrogen (estradiol) typically increases. A healthy man usually needs to maintain a testosterone (ng/dL) to estrogen (estradiol) (pg/mL) ratio of at least 10-to-1. When this ratio falls far below 10-to-1, estrogen levels become excessively high, leading to a host of health issues. Conversely, too little estrogen can result in lack of sexual interest, fewer erections, and no libido. Extremely low estrogen levels are also detrimental to brain health, and no one likes experiencing brain fog.

Low estrogen levels do not only occur naturally. Sometimes they arise from patients taking aromatase inhibitors for too long without a doctor checking their estrogen (estradiol) levels. While aromatase inhibitors effectively reduce estrogen numbers and the conversion of testosterone to estrogen, careful monitoring is necessary to prevent estrogen levels from becoming too low. This is where DIM comes into play—it lowers estrogen levels but won't push them too low.

ESTROGEN ANSWERS FOR MEN

The optimization of estrogen levels in men typically goes hand in hand with their testosterone levels. These two hormones are linked: raising testosterone levels often results in a rise in estrogen levels, while decreasing testosterone levels usually leads to a reduction in estrogen levels. The goal is for at least a 10-to-1 ratio of testosterone (ng/dL) to estrogen (pg/mL).

When men start using testosterone cream, shots, or pellets, some of the testosterone aromatizes, or converts, to estrogen. Some men have excessive aromatization, especially older men and men who are obese. Remember, the normal range for estrogen (estradiol) in men is 20–70 pg/mL. When optimizing estradiol numbers in men, I recommend aiming for estradiol levels of 20–40 pg/mL (and ideally 20–30 pg/mL). To stay in the estradiol hormone health zone, men will need to take DIM (150 milligrams once or twice a day). It is the safest way to lower estrogen without the fear of going too low.

For men who suspect they might be experiencing symptoms of either low or high estrogen and haven't had their levels checked, it's advisable to request blood work to measure their estradiol level. This will give them and their doctor the necessary information to determine the best course of treatment. Fortunately, it's usually pretty easy to manage estrogen levels in men.

While it might be surprising that men need to monitor their estrogen levels, it's something to be mindful of. In a way it's like checking for blind spots while driving. These spots might not be dangerous in and of themselves, but when you need to take action, the blind spots are suddenly very important.

Even though estrogen is a minor player, it can make a big impact if it falls outside the normal range. Armed with this knowledge, you're well-equipped to keep it in check.

TESTOSTERONE ANSWERS FOR MEN

From a biological perspective, testosterone is what makes a man. It is primarily produced in the testes but also in the adrenal glands. Most importantly, testosterone helps increase muscle mass, strength, and stamina, and it aids in fat burning. It also protects the brain, helps improve memory, helps prevent and reverse depression and irritability, decreases inflammation throughout the body, boosts energy, prevents frailty, and helps maintain a good sex drive and strong, healthy erections.

Every doctor who uses bioidentical hormone replacement therapy can tell stories of patients who suddenly went from a state of illness to one of health in one area or another. Some of these stories are astonishing because the improvements are so drastic, but that is the power of hormones at work in our bodies.

This is especially true of testosterone. It is the hormone with the most mental, emotional, and physical health benefits. It boosts energy and decreases inflammation and, usually, chronic pain. Without sufficient testosterone, our bodies pay an incredible price.

I call it the "home run hormone," as optimizing testosterone levels in men is like flipping all the essential switches in the body, igniting a healing process, especially when combined with a healthy keto or Mediterranean-keto diet. (See appendix A.)

Unfortunately, from the age of thirty-five onward, men experience an annual decline in testosterone production by 1 percent, and some sources suggest it might even be as high as 5 percent. If we use a conservative estimate of 1 percent per year, that still breaks down to a 10 percent testosterone loss per decade. Whether it's 1 percent or 5 percent, that's too much. Men need their testosterone.

Considering this gradual annual loss of testosterone, most men will begin seeing symptoms of low testosterone around the age of fifty. Add in factors like obesity, prediabetes, type 2 diabetes, nutritional deficiencies, chronic stress, medications, illnesses, diet, increased exposure to endocrine disruptors, and lack of physical activity, and the rate of testosterone loss speeds up exponentially.

Men need to be fully aware of how their bodies are changing as they age. Benjamin Franklin's old axiom "An ounce of prevention is worth a pound of cure" could not be more fitting than when it comes to testosterone. And since millions of men in the United States—half of all men over the age of fifty—may suffer from low testosterone, that makes it something men cannot and should not ignore.[1]

THE TESTOSTERONE HEALTH ZONE FOR MEN

Optimizing testosterone levels positively impacts a myriad of diseases and symptoms. If you're battling some of the symptoms and diseases linked to low or suboptimal testosterone, it is time to boost your testosterone levels to what they were when you were in your twenties.

What can you expect? In all likelihood, you'll experience a substantial improvement in your overall health, energy, and zest for life! The hormone health zone is frequently where symptoms and diseases lessen—and sometimes completely disappear. It is also where countless individuals reclaim their lives. Men, it's imperative that you know your total testosterone and free testosterone numbers. Here are the standard ranges for both.

Total testosterone ranges in men

According to LabCorp, its recommended range for men (over age eighteen) for total testosterone is 150–916 ng/dL. A few years ago it was 348–1197, but LabCorp recently lowered it. Another lab, Quest Diagnostics, has a similar range for total testosterone: 250–1100 ng/dL. When men optimize their total testosterone (pushed to the upper range of normal) to the levels they were at when they were in their twenties, total testosterone numbers will be closer to 500–1100 ng/dL.

Any man "in range" with a total testosterone number that is low or suboptimal (250–500 ng/dL) is most likely going to have negative symptoms or is developing those symptoms. A man's body needs more testosterone than the lower end of these ranges can afford. Remember, the symptoms mean more than the range does, so if you have some of the symptoms of low testosterone in your body, there is a reason for it.

Some men need their testosterone optimized even higher, to 750–1100 ng/dL, to eliminate most or all low testosterone symptoms. Unfortunately, men's testosterone levels are getting lower and lower, and labs will continue to lower the normal levels of testosterone because reference ranges are made by collecting results from a large population and determining the mean testosterone levels and the standard deviation.

Free testosterone ranges in men

The same lab companies recommend these ranges for free testosterone in men. Quest Diagnostics calculates free testosterone levels based on total testosterone, sex hormone binding globulin (SHBG), and albumin whereas LabCorp uses a direct immunoassay method with a much different reference range than Quest's:

LabCorp:

- age twenty to twenty-nine: 9.3–26.5 pg/mL
- age thirty to thirty-nine: 8.7–25.1 pg/mL
- age forty to forty-nine: 6.8–21.5 pg/mL
- age fifty to fifty-nine: 7.2–24.0 pg/mL
- over age fifty-nine: 6.6–18.1 pg/mL

Quest Diagnostics:

- age eighteen to sixty-nine: 46–224 pg/mL
- age seventy to eighty-nine: 6–73 pg/mL

Optimized free testosterone levels will look more like this:

- LabCorp—free testosterone for men: 15–26.5 pg/mL

- Quest Diagnostics—free testosterone for men: 125–224 pg/mL

The concentration of free testosterone is usually very low and usually less than 2 percent of the total testosterone concentration. Remember, the free testosterone is the active testosterone. Approximately 60 percent of total testosterone is bound to sex hormone binding globulin (SHBG), and once bound, it cannot be released and used inside cells. About 38 percent of testosterone is bound to albumin[2] and can become free testosterone again if supplemented with adequate DIM, usually 150 milligrams twice a day.

Again, most men in the lower-to-suboptimal range of testosterone are really going to be symptomatic. But when free testosterone and total testosterone are brought into optimal levels, amazing transformations take place. For example, when it comes to protection from heart disease, it was found that cardiovascular risks dropped dramatically when total testosterone levels were optimized above 550 ng/dL.[3]

When you were twenty-five, you probably weren't concerned about cholesterol, heart health, depression, sexual function, memory issues, muscle deterioration, or even your weight. You were likely too busy enjoying life! Optimizing hormone levels, particularly testosterone, has the potential to rekindle much of the same zest for life, health, disease prevention, vitality, strength, and hope you once enjoyed.

TESTS AND TREATMENT PLANS

Only when men reach a point where they can no longer ignore their symptoms (we men are masters at ignoring symptoms until they become glaringly apparent) will they typically seek medical attention. Ideally, a man's doctor will be proficient in bioidentical hormone replacement therapy.

If you have trouble finding a doctor who practices bioidentical hormone replacement therapy, you can find doctors online. Appendix B includes a list of websites that can guide you to doctors knowledgeable in bioidentical hormones.

Starting with the right tests is critical. Many doctors, even those who do not practice hormone replacement therapy, will help you get the hormonal lab tests you need. The right lab tests will likely uncover the root cause of your symptoms. Low levels of total and free testosterone are the major culprits behind so many symptoms, and it is safe to say, "I'm experiencing many symptoms of low testosterone." (Of course, your doctor will order the lab tests.) Furthermore, if either your total or free testosterone is low, the other is often low as well.

In total, I recommend the following hormone tests:

- total testosterone
- free testosterone
- TSH
- TPO antibodies
- rT3

- SHBG
- estradiol
- PSA
- free T3 level

I also check a complete blood count, a comprehensive metabolic panel, a lipid panel, a hemoglobin A1c, a 25OHD$_3$ (vitamin D$_3$) level, an hs-CRP (high-sensitivity C-reactive protein), a B$_{12}$ level, and a urinalysis.

Men have several different options for testosterone replacement therapy.

Sublingual tabs

There is no natural testosterone that you can take in pill form except sublingual testosterone tabs, or troches, prepared at a compounding pharmacy. These tabs are taken by placing one under the tongue—or even better, between the lower lip and gum—two to three times per day. Taking testosterone orally (not sublingually) usually elevates liver enzymes and may cause a drug-induced hepatitis. That's why I recommend the creams, gels, shots (injections), and pellets as the preferred ways to administer testosterone.

Creams and gels

Transdermal creams and gels are the most common form of testosterone therapy. The dosage is usually 50–200 milligrams of testosterone in 0.5–1 mL of cream applied to the skin behind the knee or antecubital fossa (area of the forearm that is hairless, where blood is often drawn) once a day. The optimal spots for applying the cream are the back of the knee, where it is hairless, and rotating sides, or the antecubital fossa. Behind the knee is preferable since it is much less likely to be transferred to children or your wife by touch. Men often prefer using a cream to raise their testosterone levels if possible, as it's a painless method. While shots and pellets effectively raise testosterone, they can be more costly and more painful. Some men hate injections and minor surgical procedures such as pellets. Testosterone creams offer better absorption through the skin compared to gels. They also moisturize the skin and do not cause dryness like alcohol-based gels. (Both creams and gels can inadvertently transfer testosterone to children and women, causing masculinizing effects.) Creams may also raise dihydrotestosterone (DHT) levels more than injections and pellets. Elevated DHT levels can trigger male pattern baldness, prostate enlargement, and acne. Additionally, creams and gels can increase estrogen levels. Although shots and pellets are usually the primary way to get testosterone levels into the optimal range, the new cream base (Atrevis) delivers testosterone through the skin by using several naturally derived permeation enhancers. It's now possible to optimize testosterone levels without resorting to shots or pellets, which is particularly good news for patients who dislike those methods. If you do apply your testosterone cream to the antecubital fossa, do not do so on the day you have your blood drawn. It can cause a falsely high serum testosterone level. Also, some men choose to apply smaller amounts of testosterone cream (5–25 milligrams) daily to the perianal area, which is absorbed much better. For these individuals, I prescribe testosterone in Vanicream. A drawback is this tends to raise DHT levels. More on this later.

Shots

More and more, injections are becoming less painful and easier to give. Their effects can last for several days, so just one or two shots per week are usually enough. Nowadays, these shots can be administered subcutaneously using very fine needles, and they can be injected into the lateral thigh, buttock, or deltoid muscle. These injections are usually almost painless and rarely result in bruising. Some compounding pharmacies will even preload the syringes for you, eliminating the need for measuring. Regardless of the method, shots remain highly effective for optimizing testosterone levels.

Pellets

While typically more expensive than alternative methods, pellets are by far the easiest and most effective way to raise your testosterone levels. With just five to ten 200 milligram pellets implanted every six months, you can essentially put the matter out of your mind. These pellets, roughly the size of a grain of rice, are inserted in the hip area and the dosage is based on your body weight and testosterone level. While it is a minor surgical procedure, it's generally quick, easy, and usually painless.

OTHER FACTORS THAT AFFECT TESTOSTERONE THERAPY

In addition to testing the hormones you want to optimize, always remember to keep an eye on the other factors that can adversely affect the testosterone therapy. For men that includes the following:

Estradiol

Men on testosterone therapy may also be elevating their estradiol levels. Keeping the estradiol level between 20 and 40 pg/mL is good (20–30 pg/mL is ideal).[4]

SHBG

Approximately 60 percent of testosterone is bound to SHBG in healthy young men.[5] When testosterone is bound to SHBG, it can no longer be used by the body. Elderly men usually have much higher SHBG levels and decreased levels of free testosterone, which is the testosterone that can be used by the body. Men, if your SHBG is high, you will probably need a higher dose of testosterone to optimize your free testosterone, or else you could have a high normal testosterone level and still have numerous symptoms of low testosterone because the majority of your testosterone is bound by SHBG. If you have low testosterone symptoms and high normal total testosterone levels, be sure to check your SHBG and free testosterone levels.

DHT

Testosterone is converted to DHT—which I call "testosterone's nasty little cousin"—by the enzyme 5-alpha-reductase. DHT is very masculinizing and causes your voice to lower at puberty and hair to grow on your groin, face, and chest. It's also the main cause of male pattern baldness, enlargement of the prostate, and acne. Keeping an eye on DHT is recommended if you are developing these symptoms. It can usually be controlled by putting testosterone cream on a hairless area (such as behind the knee), decreasing the dose of testosterone, changing to pellets, or using herbs such as saw palmetto or beta-sitosterol or meds such as finasteride or dutasteride to minimize conversion.

DIM

For lowering estradiol, taking diindolylmethane (DIM), a natural supplement made from broccoli, will usually help lower estradiol levels that may try to creep up. This is especially true for men as they age.[6] Taking 150–200 milligrams of DIM once or twice a day is usually sufficient to keep estradiol levels in check. Some men may need to take it three times a day, and very rarely some men need a low dose of Arimidex (usually 0.5–1 milligram once or twice a week), which is another estrogen blocker, or aromatase inhibitor. (See appendix B.)

TESTOSTERONE LEVELS ARE DROPPING

At this point you might be thinking, "How do I know if I need testosterone replacement therapy?"

That is a valid question. The answer is going to be based on your symptoms and your needs, but if you are looking for a number, you can call 500 ng/dL your cutoff point. If your total testosterone number is less than 500 ng/dL and you are beginning to notice some symptoms of low testosterone—including decreased strength, decreased stamina and endurance, decreased libido, loss of early morning erection, fatigue, and increased irritability (see page 170 of *Dr. Colbert's Hormone Health Zone* for a complete list)—you have your answer. At that point I would suggest you start testosterone replacement therapy.

This applies whether you are thirty-nine or ninety-nine years old unless you want more children. Then you would need to get a prescription for Clomid (clomiphene citrate) or hCG (human chorionic gonadotropin) injections. (Over-the-counter testosterone boosters can also be helpful.) Testosterone can lower sperm counts and should not be used in younger men wanting to have children.

You do not need to go through life or finish out your life battling the countless symptoms of low testosterone. Everyone else might, but you don't have to! Across the board, testosterone levels are dropping in American men[7] and have been for decades.

Furthermore, consider the increased prevalence of heart disease, obesity, type 2 diabetes, sarcopenia, osteoporosis, dementia, Parkinson's, and

Alzheimer's. These and many other diseases are increasing exactly in sync with the decline of our testosterone levels.

As we've discussed extensively in this book, there are myriad reasons why our testosterone levels are plummeting. For most people it's a combination of excess weight, nutritional deficiencies, chronic stress, medications, diseases, diet, hormone disruptors, and aging. Chances are your testosterone levels are not at their optimal state.

If you're using statin drugs to lower your cholesterol (likely at your doctor's recommendation), there's almost no chance your testosterone levels are in a healthy range. As previously mentioned, testosterone is made from cholesterol in your body, so decreasing cholesterol often leads to a decrease in testosterone levels as well. Fortunately, as you already know, optimized testosterone levels typically lower the bad cholesterol and increase the good cholesterol in your body.

If you are fighting obesity, the increased fat around the internal organs increases the conversion of testosterone to estrogen.[8] That means your body continues to produce excessive estrogen, exacerbating obesity and giving rise to an array of negative symptoms and diseases. Diet, exercise, and testosterone replacement therapy are crucial to break this detrimental cycle.

If the goal is to avoid ending up in a nursing home, optimize your testosterone levels. Allowing muscle to turn to fat is a sure way to lose your independence. Keep your testosterone levels up and exercise. I have some eighty-five-year-old patients who can do a three-minute plank! Most people can hardly do it for sixty seconds. Maintain your muscle and you maintain your overall health.

Unfortunately, the trend toward lowering testosterone is only going to continue, and we are doing nothing as a society to stop it. The only defense is your own defense. You determine what kind of life you'll have in the future by the choices you make today.

PART IV:
SAFEGUARD YOUR BRAIN

CHAPTER 15

PRESERVE YOUR BRAIN VITALITY

P EOPLE RECOIL WHEN the words *Alzheimer's* or *dementia* are used. They step back, and usually fear grips their hearts as well as their minds. But despite the rampant trends, news, and statistics, there is hope. There are answers out there. No magic pill makes everything go away, but proven steps, protocols, health measures, and options can truly help you slow, manage, stop, or reverse Alzheimer's and dementia. If you are on this journey for yourself or friends or family, I encourage you not to delay. Time is of the essence, so jump right in and apply all that you learn here. If you are seeking a fuller picture of what contributes to cognitive decline and how to combat it, dive into my book *Dr. Colbert's Healthy Brain Zone.*

GET YOUR BLOOD WORK

You can't form an effective plan if you don't know where you're starting. In the fight against Alzheimer's and dementia, the starting point is knowing your numbers. That's why I usually recommend patients begin with a full-panel blood test to figure out where they are currently. Then when you get the results back, you will know more clearly which areas need to be worked on.

I've provided a complete list of tests and your target values for each test in appendix B. Please photocopy this list to show the doctor who orders your blood work, and then use it to compare the target values with your blood work reports. If you have a positive ApoE4 gene test (the Alzheimer's gene), it will be especially important for you to achieve the target values for blood work and trophic factors from the list in appendix B.

Looking at the target values in the appendix without your blood work will be a little confusing, but trust me, it will make much more sense when you can compare your results with these numbers. Knowledge is your power because the more you know, the better equipped you are to make the right health decisions for your current and long-term needs.

GET OTHER TESTING

As I said, I believe everyone needs a full-panel blood test as a first step. That's because, regardless of our genetics, all of us need to monitor those numbers throughout our lives to prevent, repair, or reverse the damage our choices and environment can cause. Beyond that, most should want to know their genetic risk level for developing Alzheimer's. If that's you, I strongly recommend getting the ApoE genetic (genotype) test and following the dietary and lifestyle recommendations.

The ApoE4 gene gives instructions for making a protein called apolipoprotein E4. This protein then joins with fats to form lipoproteins. The lipoproteins then package cholesterol and other fats and transport them through the blood. If you have the ApoE4 gene, you are at the greatest risk for Alzheimer's and dementia, as well as heart attack and stroke.

An ApoE gene test at a lab (with your doctor's order for it) will give you your results. I request this all the time for my patients. It is the strongest known genetic risk factor for Alzheimer's disease. You can't remove the gene from your body, but you can do a lot to prevent Alzheimer's and dementia even if you have the gene.

If you've noticed early signs of cognitive decline and want conclusive evidence of what you're dealing with, then consider getting a brain scan or a MoCA test (Montreal Cognitive Assessment test at www.mocatest. org). Many physicians perform the thirty-question MoCA test in their offices, as I do, to help detect cognitive impairment. If you answer eighteen to twenty-five questions correctly, that indicates mild cognitive impairment. If you get ten to seventeen answers correct, you have moderate cognitive impairment. If you get fewer than ten questions correct, then there is severe cognitive impairment.

MoCA

In Alzheimer's cases, a positron emission tomography (PET) scan will show a consistent pattern of decreased glucose uptake, especially in your hippocampus, which is located near your temples. The hippocampus is where information is stored temporarily before the brain processes it and moves it to your permanent memory.

EVALUATE YOUR TEST RESULTS

The PET scan of the brain is optional, but not the blood work. Why? Because you can do everything you need to do to fight Alzheimer's and dementia with the blood tests I recommend in appendix B. Once you have your blood work results, you'll want to compare them to the target values I've listed in the appendix.

Your blood work results will determine your plan. Then you will know what steps from the following chapters are required to slow, manage, stop, or reverse memory loss and put you in the Healthy Brain Zone.

For the rest of this chapter, I'll highlight a few key blood test results to look for, and the rest of the chapters of this book will outline the twelve steps you need to follow to correct these numbers and put yourself on the path to the Healthy Brain Zone.

A1c and glucose levels

One of the most common dementogens is sweeteners and sugars (from sweets, carbs, and starches). Your hemoglobin A1c numbers will tell the story: an A1c of 5.6 or lower is normal—however, if you are having memory loss, your A1c should be 5.3 or less—5.7–6.4 is prediabetic, and 6.5 or higher is diabetic. About 40 percent of the adult US population is diabetic or prediabetic. People with type 2 diabetes may be two times more likely to develop Alzheimer's.[1] So if you have type 2 diabetes or are prediabetic, now is the time to act.

Even if your A1c and glucose levels are normal, keep an eye on your waistline. Those with more belly fat have an almost three times greater risk of dementia than less-overweight people.[2] In light of this, if you are overweight, losing weight is an important part of your action plan.

But don't lose too much! You need to maintain a minimum body mass index of 18.5 if you're a woman and 19.0 if you're a man under age sixty-five, but it should be higher if you are over sixty-five. Losing too much weight increases the risk of sarcopenia (loss of muscle) and osteopenia (loss of bone). People with these diseases have an increased risk of cognitive decline.[3]

As discussed in part 2 of this book, I recommend a healthy keto diet for weight loss and then transitioning to a Mediterranean-keto diet as a lifestyle.

Cholesterol levels

Your blood work results will include your cholesterol numbers. Everyone is told to lower their cholesterol, but it is worth noting that if you push it below 150, you may be starving your brain and increasing your risk of brain atrophy.[4] A cholesterol level between 150 and 200 is best for your brain.

Chronic infections and inflammation

If your blood test shows that you have an elevated hs-CRP that doesn't come down, this may be an indicator of a chronic infection or Lyme disease. All chronic infections increase the risk of cognitive decline, whether you know you have them or not. Standard blood work will not usually confirm if you have chronic infections, which is why I recommend specific blood work for Lyme or Lyme coinfections, antibodies to herpes simplex virus 1, and more. Please compare your results with the target values in appendix B.

Inflammation also causes cognitive decline. Remember, type 1 Alzheimer's is usually associated with elevated inflammatory markers, including an elevated C-reactive protein, an increase in tumor necrosis factor, an increase in interleukin-6 (IL-6), or an increase in nuclear factor kappa B (NFKB). It is also associated with a decrease in the albumin-to-globulin ratio.

Don't Put It Off!

These key lab tests, along with indicators of suboptimal nutrient and hormone levels and toxins in the body, will paint the full picture of where you're starting. And the time to start is now! A list of the most important blood tests is in appendix B.

Please don't delay. The first phase of Alzheimer's and dementia is when communication between brain cells is jammed, connections are lost, and cells die. The best time to take action is now. Beware of anyone, especially a doctor, who tells you to wait, see how it goes, and come back next year. When most people are diagnosed with Alzheimer's or dementia, it has already been affecting them for fifteen to twenty years![5] The earlier you take action, the better off you are.

Never forget that developing Alzheimer's and dementia is not inevitable and those exhibiting signs of memory loss are not hopeless cases. The scary statistics, such as the rate of new Alzheimer's cases doubling every five years from age sixty-five to ninety,[6] are based on people who are doing nothing to prevent, slow, manage, stop, or reverse memory loss.

They are not taking action, but you are. Every step is a positive movement, moving toward a better and stronger brain. Every step, even if it feels small and insignificant, is a step in the right direction. You are taking action, so be encouraged. You are on the right road!

CHAPTER 16

NUTRITIONAL NEUROPROTECTION

THE BEST DIET to prevent, slow, manage, stop, or reverse Alzheimer's and dementia is, without question, a healthy keto diet. The Mediterranean diet comes in second. Therefore, I recommend starting with a healthy keto diet and then shifting over later (if you want) to a Mediterranean-keto diet.

I consider the Mediterranean-keto diet easier to maintain than a healthy keto diet. Both are incredibly healthy options and the best diets anywhere, but I always recommend that people start with a healthy keto diet, especially if they have any symptoms of memory loss, mild cognitive impairment, or mild, moderate, or severe Alzheimer's disease.

The keto diet is a low-carb, high-fat, and moderate-protein eating plan, but many people on the keto diet are following an unhealthy version. The healthy keto diet that I recommend in this book and in my book *Beyond Keto* includes a lot of healthy fats from fatty fish, such as wild salmon, sardines, wild mackerel, wild herring, and anchovies, which are high in omega-3 fats and very low in mercury.

My book *Beyond Keto* goes into greater detail and is a must-read if you embark upon a keto diet. It also has the unique benefit of combining the best of keto with the best of the Mediterranean diet in one book. The great thing is that the benefits of a Mediterranean-keto diet align with the list of things we need to do to reduce the buildup of amyloid plaque in the brain.

These benefits match what you need to fight Alzheimer's and dementia. There are many more reasons to be on a healthy keto diet, but the fact that such a diet prevents, slows, manages, stops, or reverses Alzheimer's and dementia is amazing.

Of course, you are the one who decides what to eat and makes any diet a habit. I've had patients in the worst situations (diagnosed with cancer, chronic diseases, dementia, Alzheimer's, and more) reap amazing results when they chose to get on a healthy keto diet. It works incredibly well.

Prevention is always the best option, but sometimes we have no choice and need to fix, repair, or reverse a health condition, and thankfully the body can do just that!

With Alzheimer's and dementia, people are most often in the fixing phase, and I understand that, but I hope someday there will be more people in the prevention phase. That is where we all need to be.

FEED YOUR BODY, BENEFIT YOUR BRAIN

Feeding your body the correct food will always benefit your brain. That's a direct effect, but it's also the intended result because we are in a position now as a country (and world) where we must act without delay.

4. *72 percent or higher dark chocolate that is low in sugar and high in flavanols*

5. *sardines, wild salmon, and other high-fat, low-mercury wild fish*

6. *avocados*

7. *pastured, organic eggs*

8. *walnuts, almonds, pecans, and macadamia nuts*

9. *curry sauce full of curcumin, or turmeric*

10. *kale*

A healthy keto diet also contains a lot of healthy cold-pressed oils, such as extra-virgin olive oil, avocado oil, macadamia nut oil, almond oil, and tahini, along with sesame seeds, avocados, nuts, and seeds. Organic is always best.

Less than 10 percent of your fat intake, or about 1 teaspoon to 1 tablespoon or less a day, should come from saturated fats such as grass-fed butter, grass-fed ghee, coconut oil, MCT oil, and other saturated fats.

While on a healthy keto diet, you burn fat in addition to burning ketones for fuel. That means a breakthrough for many patients because fat (especially belly fat) is what is pushing them toward Alzheimer's and dementia.

These ketones (produced in your liver) are almost all used for fuel (more than 80 percent), and the rest are exhaled or passed in your urine.[1]

Are these ketones good for your brain? Absolutely! The fact is,

- ketones give the brain more energy than a typical glucose-derived diet can, which improves cognitive function in Alzheimer's patients;[2]

- ketones decrease Parkinson's disease symptoms by 43 percent after just one month;[3]

- ketones fuel up to 75 percent of the brain's energy needs; while the brain still needs a small amount of glucose, when someone has Alzheimer's or diabetes, the brain no longer uses glucose effectively due to insulin resistance; however, ketones can compensate for this brain fuel deficit.[4]

Once your body is used to eating less sugar, fewer carbs, more healthy fats, and moderate amounts of protein, insulin resistance, which is one of the hallmarks of Alzheimer's and dementia, will improve and may eventually resolve.

DR. COLBERT'S BRAIN SMOOTHIE

» ½ cup frozen organic blueberries or strawberries or other berry or mixed berries

» ½–1 cup triple-washed organic kale

» ¼–½ teaspoon stevia

» 8 ounces filtered or pure water

Blend until smooth.

As is done with a healthy keto diet, feeding your body the right food fuels your brain. Quite often the brain is the afterthought. It's expected to keep up and do its job. But based on national and global trends, the brain eventually cannot perform as intended. It is unable to. And this takes us right back to the recent findings that Alzheimer's and dementia are the results of a brain trying to cope in an unfriendly, toxic, starved environment.

The answer? Simply this: give your brain the fuel it needs! A healthy keto diet will do just that. And because a healthy keto or Mediterranean-keto diet (if you choose to shift over to it) feeds your body exactly what it needs to prevent, slow, manage, stop, or reverse Alzheimer's and dementia, you now know your next step.

As you know, doctors prescribe medications that can and do provide a temporary boost to the brain, but medications do not and cannot replace a healthy diet. As always, anything less than a fix is just a bandage approach. Once your healthy diet is in place, there are things you can do to improve memory, boost mental energy, support neural health, clean out cellular debris, and much more. All this helps protect your brain from Alzheimer's and dementia.

Twenty-Five Ways to Fuel Your Brain

So many different supplements, activities, nutrients, habits, and foods help support, strengthen, and benefit your brain that it's impossible to list them all here. The existence of such a wide variety of brain boosters shows just how susceptible the brain is to outside forces. Some of those listed here are big, and some are small, but they all combine to make an impact.

The converse is also true. It's easy to damage your brain by making small, unhealthy choices on a daily basis. Multiply the many bad influences over years and decades, and you have the Alzheimer's and dementia epidemic we face today!

But you know better. Once you are standing on the foundation of a healthy diet, here are several brain boosters you can put into action for additional fuel for your brain.

1. Consume healthy fats.

Healthy fats help fuel your brain.[5] These include extra-virgin olive oil, avocados and avocado oil, coconut oil (in small amounts), flaxseed oil, almond butter, raw nuts (almonds, macadamia, pecans, walnuts), seeds (chia, pine, Salba, hemp), and MCT oil or powder (in moderation). These do not include trans fats or unhealthy oils such as soybean, corn, canola, peanut, sunflower, safflower, cottonseed, or palm kernel.[6]

2. Sharpen your focus.

You can sharpen and improve your focus with practice, sufficient sleep, exercise, caffeine, gotu kola (100–500 milligrams once or twice a day), vitamin B_5 (100–200 milligrams per day), MCT oil (½–1 teaspoon once or twice a day), and acetyl L-Carnitine (500 milligrams twice daily).[7]

3. Increase your BDNF.

Brain-derived neurotrophic factor (BDNF) is a protein that helps your brain grow new neurons, helps existing neurons, and encourages synapse formation. Alzheimer's patients have decreased BDNF levels.[8] Exercise, raising testosterone and estradiol hormone levels, intermittent fasting, and ketones from being on a healthy keto diet will raise your BDNF levels. So will a whole coffee fruit extract (WCFE) supplement. I recommend 100–200 milligrams twice a day of WCFE. Also, 25 milligrams twice a day of tropoflavin (also known as 7,8 dihydroxyflavone) increases BDNF, and the mushroom lion's mane increases BDNF. More on this later.

4. Protect with DHEA.

DHEA protects the neurons in your brain. Many people, especially those over fifty, may need to take DHEA to keep their brains safe. My recommendation: micronized DHEA 10 milligrams once or twice daily for women and 25 milligrams once or twice daily for men.

5. Get more DHA.

The brain cannot make DHA but needs it for cognition, brain support, and neurotransmitters. About 90 percent of omega-3 fatty acids in the brain are DHA, and DHA is one of the main fats for synapses.[9] Look for omega-3 (fish oil) with at least a 1-to-1 ratio or more of DHA to EPA. Fish is an excellent source of DHA. Choose fish high in omega-3 but low in mercury and toxins, such as SMASH fish: sardines, mackerel, anchovies, wild salmon, and herring. Vegans and vegetarians are often woefully low in DHA, which is bad for the brain.

The truth is that most people are not getting enough DHA in their diet. How much DHA do people need? I recommend 1,000 milligrams two times per day. I personally take about 2,000 milligrams a day. The FDA claims that omega-3 supplements containing EPA and DHA are safe if doses don't exceed 3,000 milligrams per day. The European Food Safety Authority says supplementing up to 5,000 milligrams of EPA and DHA daily is safe.[10] If you have the ApoE4 gene, you need even more DHA. Vegans can take algal oil, which is vegan and has a very high ratio of DHA to EPA.

6. Support brain health with Synapsin nasal spray.

This nasal spray is a blend of ginsenoside Rg3, nicotinamide riboside, and methylcobalamin, which is the active form of vitamin B_{12}. It supports neurological health and cognitive health. Ask your doctor for a prescription. I prescribe this commonly for patients with any memory problem—mild, moderate, or severe. Rg3 is isolated from Panax ginseng and is neuroprotective. Nicotinamide riboside provides increased NAD+ levels for neurons, which also has neuroprotective effects and improves mitochondria metabolism in the neurons. Methylcobalamin lowers homocysteine levels. High levels of this toxic amino acid contribute to brain degeneration and arterial plaque, among other things.

7. Take lion's mane for better memory.

Taking lion's mane (a mushroom) has been found to help improve cognitive function and prevent deterioration, among many other health benefits.[11] This supplement is available in most health food stores. One of my patients with diabetes had a stroke and lost his memory. He started taking lion's mane 250–500 milligrams three times per day and experienced a full return of his memory! Lion's mane stimulates the production of both nerve growth factor (NGF) and brain-derived neurotrophic factor (BDNF).

8. Heal leaky gut with bone broth.

Bone broth has glutamine, an amino acid that helps heal leaky gut.[12] You can make your own bone broth. Adjust as needed, but one simple recipe includes 2 pounds of pastured animal bones in 2 quarts of water. Add salt, onions, garlic, 1 tablespoon of vinegar, and other spices. Slow-cook or pressure-cook. Drink a cup daily, freeze extra if you made a large batch, and use in meals.

9. Curb inflammation with curcumin.

Curcumin, the active ingredient in turmeric, is anti-inflammatory and an antioxidant, inhibiting free radicals.[13] It binds to amyloid plaque, which helps your body expel it, thus decreasing the buildup of amyloid plaque in your brain. Combine curcumin with black pepper and it increases its bioavailability by 2,000 percent.[14] It also helps with memory function. In one study, 90 milligrams given to random participants for eighteen months increased memory function by 28 percent for those between the ages of fifty and ninety.[15]

10. Maintain brain health with vitamin D.

Vitamin D turns on more than nine hundred genes! It helps create and maintain brain synapses.[16] Found in fatty fish (sardines and salmon), egg yolks, mushrooms, and cod liver oil, vitamin D is often referred to as "the sunshine vitamin" because exposing our skin to sunlight increases its production. You do not want to be deficient in this vitamin, for those with cognitive decline usually have low levels of vitamin D. It is readily available as a supplement. The goal is to bring your vitamin D_3 level (or $25OHD_3$ level) to 55–80 ng/mL.

11. Boost key hormones.

Boosting your hormones, especially pregnenolone, DHEA, testosterone, estradiol, and thyroid, has been found to support the brain in many ways.[17]

12. Lower homocysteine level.

Ideally, your homocysteine level should be 7 or lower if you have the ApoE4 gene, which is the Alzheimer's gene, but initially aim for a level less than 10. A high level contributes to osteoporosis, brain degeneration, Alzheimer's, and plaque in your arteries and is a sign of inflammation and loss of synapse-supporting nutrients.[18] Recently a patient brought in lab work I had ordered to check her homocysteine level. It was 17, which, according to the lab, was normal. Regardless of what the lab considered normal, I knew her homocysteine level of 17 was quite high. (A homocysteine level of 19–20 is considered extremely high and is associated with memory loss.) But unfortunately most doctors don't know this and would have thought her homocysteine level was normal.

This toxic amino acid can be lowered with the right amounts of the following: 20 milligrams per day of vitamin B_6 (in its active form as pyridoxal 5'-phosphate), 1–5 milligrams per day of folic acid (in its active form as methyl tetrahydrofolate), 1 milligram per day of vitamin B_{12} (in its active form as methylcobalamin), and 500 milligrams twice a day of betaine (trimethyl glycine). If someone has a major MTHFR gene mutation, they will need the higher dose of methyl tetrahydrofolate.

Vegetarians often have high homocysteine levels because they do not eat meat, which contains vitamin B$_{12}$. I recommend the active forms of these B vitamins. MTHFR mutation affects about 40 percent of the population and is associated with decreased folic acid metabolism and decreased methylation.[19]

These patients are also at risk of higher homocysteine levels, memory loss, and brain degeneration. If you have a MTHFR gene mutation, you are at a higher risk of memory loss. I recommend the MTHFR gene test to determine if you have a MTHFR gene mutation and that you check your homocysteine level. (See appendix B for supplement recommendations for those with the MTHFR gene mutation.)

13. Heal your gut.

Without a healthy gut, it will be a very slow and difficult process (if not impossible) to prevent, slow, manage, stop, or reverse Alzheimer's and dementia. Having a healthy gut is vital! Some even call the gut the "second brain," which shows how important it is.[20] A healthy gut is one of the best defenses against Alzheimer's, dementia, and Parkinson's. Simply put, you must heal your gut. That usually begins with killing any bad bacteria. Next, you must plant good bacteria. After you repair your gut, you must avoid whatever caused your gut troubles in the first place.[21] Bone broth daily, collagen, and probiotics will also help heal your gut. See part 1 of this book and *Dr. Colbert's Healthy Gut Zone* book for steps, recipes, and more information for healing your gut.

14. Get adequate zinc.

Being deficient in zinc is common for Alzheimer's and dementia patients. Without adequate zinc, copper may build up, causing inflammation and amyloid plaque in your brain. Aim for a 1-to-1 copper-to-zinc ratio by taking zinc supplements. I suggest 15–20 milligrams of zinc per day but not more than 50 milligrams of zinc per day. Vegetarians are also often low in zinc due to their diet.

15. Increase choline.

Choline is found in egg yolks, chicken, fish, meat, and dairy. Choline is necessary for your brain because it stimulates the production of acetylcholine.[22]

Acetylcholine plays an essential role in your memory, cognition, and sleep. By prescribing Aricept, doctors are trying to raise acetylcholine levels by inhibiting the enzyme that breaks down acetylcholine. Many supplements available at health food stores will increase your acetylcholine production, including huperzine A, Bacopa, gotu kola, American ginseng, and others. DHA (from omega-3 fish oil) also increases acetylcholine.[23] Plant-based supplements are also available. I recommend alpha-GPC or citicoline 500 milligrams twice daily to increase choline and acetylcholine in the brain.

16. Boost your vitamin A (retinol).

Retinol is the active form of vitamin A, and beta-carotene is the precursor of vitamin A and is referred to as provitamin A. Everyone has heard of beta-carotene, the carotenoid vitamin A found in carrots, sweet potatoes, green leafy vegetables, and more. But the retinol vitamin A (found mostly in meat, eggs, and dairy) is important due to its protection against Alzheimer's and dementia. Supplements of vitamin A retinol are available at health food stores. I recommend 900 micrograms of RAE (retinol activity equivalents), or 3,000 IU, for men and 700 micrograms RAE (2,333 IU) for women each day. I personally take vitamin A every day. One microgram RAE is equivalent to 1 microgram retinol.

17. Enjoy some java.

Coffee helps you wake up; improves mood; boosts learning; aids recall; helps protect against Parkinson's, cancer, liver disease, and memory loss; and is good for your brain.[24] I recommend no more than four 8 oz. cups of coffee per day with the last cup before 3 p.m. Drinking more than 32 ounces of coffee a day can increase homocysteine levels by 20 percent.[25]

18. Get your sleep.

Sleep helps your brain catalog and store information; consolidate, declutter, and store memories properly; and clear out old cells, toxic debris, and amyloid plaque. All this directly decreases your risk of Alzheimer's and dementia. I recommend seven to eight hours of sleep each night.

19. Get more active.

Exercise fuels your brain like nothing else. You don't need to run marathons; just being active is the best defense against cognitive decline.[26] Exercise will boost blood flow to your brain, increase your synaptic connections, grow new neurons, keep brain cells alive, protect you from dementogens, improve your memory recall, boost your brain-derived neurotrophic factors (BDNF) production, and help remove amyloid plaque from your brain. I recommend at minimum walking three to five thousand steps a day (or twenty to thirty minutes) five times per week. The more exercise the better, so there is no maximum. It's all fuel for your brain.

20. Raise your nerve growth factor (NGF) levels.

NGF is a protein in your brain that boosts your mental capacity, primarily by providing support to cholinergic neurons in the brain, which are critical for forming memories.[27] In other words, NGF helps your brain grow, rewire, stretch, and learn as it did when you were young. I think of NGF as "Miracle-Gro for your mind." You can raise your NGF levels by taking supplements such as lion's mane mushroom, rosemary, zinc, acetyl L-carnitine (ALCAR), lithium, DHEA, and vitamin D_3. Lion's mane is typically dosed at 250 milligrams, and patients usually start with one capsule three times per day and increase the dose after a few weeks up to 500 milligrams three times per day if needed. On average, the dosage of lion's mane is 500–1500 milligrams a day. The dose of ALCAR that increases NGF is usually 500–1000 milligrams one to three times per day. (See appendix B for recommended supplements.)

21. Deal with stress.

Stress is a powerful force that will uproot, wear down, and eventually destroy neurons in your brain and decrease glucose uptake by brain cells, starving them of fuel. And if the stress is chronic, the process will usually accelerate. You must deal with your stress, for when you do, it unleashes a wave of healing to every part of your body. Exercise, laughter, prayer, relaxing, slowing down, and choosing to change are collectively productive ways to reduce the effects of stress in your life. See my *Stress Less* book for more practical information.

22. Take phosphatidylserine supplements.

Phosphatidylserine (often called Neuro PS or PS) is a nutrient found in a variety of food such as egg yolks, organ meats, dairy, green leafy vegetables, and fish. PS helps neurotransmitters, improves memory, and boosts concentration.[28] When taking PS supplements, I usually recommend 100 milligrams three times per day, and choose PS from non-GMO sunflower lecithin instead of soy lecithin.

23. Consider lithium orotate supplements.

Lithium orotate promotes a positive mental outlook, supports detoxification enzymes in the brain, and boosts neurotransmitter activity and brain-derived neurotrophic factor (BDNF).[29] Lithium is not officially a micronutrient. Lithium concentrations in water and soil can vary significantly. In the 1940s doctors started using lithium in high doses for mania. Scientists have found a link between low lithium and negative effects on cognition. A large study in Denmark found that those drinking water with lower levels of lithium had higher rates of dementia.[30] With lithium, a small amount will do. With supplements I recommend 5 milligrams of lithium orotate once or twice per day. These are available in health food stores or online. (See appendix B for recommended supplements.)

24. Increase your magnesium threonate intake.

This form of magnesium easily crosses the blood-brain barrier, improves cognitive function, protects brain cells, preserves cognitive function, and helps improve memory.[31] This supplement is available in health food stores. I recommend 2,000 milligrams of magnesium threonate at bedtime each night.

25. Don't discount the power of faith.

Andrew Newberg, MD, director of the Center for Spirituality and the Mind at the University of Pennsylvania, has studied brain scans to observe the changes in the brain that occur as a result of prayer and other religious activities. He has noted that prayer activates the brain's frontal lobe, which helps protect the brain from deterioration. He also notes that the "primitive" area of the brain is deactivated by prayer, meaning anger and stress are lessened through prayer. Other studies have found that prayer boosts your immune system and helps you live longer. I encourage you to pray and read your Bible daily to strengthen your health—physically, mentally, emotionally, and spiritually.

SUPPLEMENT YOUR BRAIN

How many people around you have a healthy diet and fuel their brains? According to national trends and statistics, not many, if any at all. But you can and should—especially if you're trying to prevent, slow, manage, stop, or reverse Alzheimer's and dementia.

As you can tell, it's easy to add extra fuel to your brain, but please don't think I'm suggesting you add all these brain fuel options to your day. That would be too much. Too much is simply too much, leading to frustration and discouragement. I recommend that you choose based on what you want, what you can afford, what fits into your day, and what makes sense for your health goals.

These are the ones I commonly recommend (specific products are listed in appendix B):

- a good multivitamin (See appendix B.)

- vitamin D_3 (Your vitamin D level should be 55–80 ng/mL.)

- supplements to balance or optimize key hormones, especially DHEA and testosterone

- methylated B vitamins, including methyl folate 1–5 milligrams daily, methylcobalamin 1 milligram daily, vitamin B_6 20 micrograms (See appendix B.)

- DHA 1,000 milligrams twice a day to lower homocysteine levels

- curcumin 1,000 milligrams twice a day (See appendix B.)

- coffee with ½ teaspoon of MCT oil powder once or twice a day

- citicoline 500 milligrams twice a day (See appendix B.)

- 7, 8 dihydroxyflavone 25 milligrams twice a day (See appendix B.)

- lithium orotate 5 milligrams twice a day (See appendix B.)

- lion's mane mushroom 500 milligrams two or three times per day (See appendix B.)

If memory is not improving, add

- Synapsin with methylcobalamin nose spray,

- Neuro Mag 3 at bedtime,

- sildenafil 50 milligrams once a day, and

- intermittent fasting for sixteen hours a day five to seven days a week.

Adding these to a healthy diet makes for the most powerful defense against Alzheimer's and dementia possible. In all you do, keep moving forward. Every step that becomes a habit is further protection for your brain. A protected brain is a healthy brain, and a healthy brain is your future!

CHAPTER 17

HEALTH ZONE PROTOCOLS
FOR BRAIN LONGEVITY

WHEN YOU KNOW the state of your brain and overall health, then you can take the necessary steps to achieve the health you want. Taking action is the whole reason for knowing how your brain works and what it takes to keep it healthy.

As you formulate your plan to improve your brain health, there are many lifestyle changes to consider. This chapter outlines three key steps that will help you maintain a healthy brain and decrease your risk of Alzheimer's and dementia to the point that it's no longer a concern. These steps will benefit everyone, because they are not only habits for brain health but for good health in general.

KEY 1: GET A GOOD NIGHT'S SLEEP

Not getting enough sleep is not only bothersome, making you feel groggy and irritable throughout the day, but it's bad for your health. Even worse, it's bad for your brain.

A lack of sleep has a pretty scary list of results:

- increased risk for Alzheimer's
- increased risk for dementia
- increased risk for heart disease
- increased risk for type 2 diabetes
- increased risk for depression
- weight gain
- slower healing

- accelerated aging
- fatigue
- weakened immune system

How much sleep does a person need? It varies with age, but it's safe to say that we all need seven to eight hours of sleep a night. Teens need eight to ten, but few of them get that much.[1]

The average American gets 6.8 hours of sleep a night.[2] That's close, but your body needs a consistent seven to eight hours of sleep each night.

Over the years, I've seen a lot of patients who, among other things, suffered from a lack of sleep. They always had the usual reasons for not being able to sleep (i.e., noise, work schedule, heat, TV on, lights on, medications, worry, stress), but some patients had less common causes for not getting the sleep they needed. If you have trouble sleeping, the protocols in this chapter will address many of these lesser known causes of sleeplessness: gut health, eating habits, and hormone balance all have an effect on your ability to sleep. Another cause to consider is sleep apnea.

CAN'T SLEEP? IT MAY BE SLEEP APNEA

Patients with sleep apnea are typically tired when they wake up, and their spouses will tell you that during the night they were gasping for air, snoring loudly, or even not breathing for ten to thirty seconds at a time. (Those are the most common signs of sleep apnea.)

As people get older and gain weight (especially those who are obese or have a large neck—seventeen inches or more for men and sixteen inches or more for women), the chances of having sleep apnea increase.

Sleep apnea starves your brain of oxygen, which is why it's so bad for your brain and causes memory loss. This makes sense, because the brain's neurons die if they don't get enough oxygen.

If you have sleep apnea or think you may have it, you need a sleep study. A simple and inexpensive pulse oximeter will tell you instantly what your oxygen levels are, and they should be 95–98 percent. Levels below 90 percent indicate low oxygen.

However, you should ideally have a sleep study. You can also assess your breathing during sleep via a wrist pulse oximeter, which has a silicone probe worn on your finger and an oxygen monitor that allows you to observe and review your oxygen data. These can be purchased online for around $100.

If you have mild sleep apnea, weight loss of more than twenty pounds or a dental or nasal device can help. But if you have more severe sleep apnea, I strongly suggest you get fitted for a CPAP machine. These machines increase your oxygen levels at night, ensuring your brain is not starved of oxygen.

For many of my patients, getting a CPAP machine improved their sleep and helped them dream again, and for many, it fixed or improved their memory-related issues.

Snap Diagnostics (snapdiagnostics.com) is one company I often recommend to patients I suspect have sleep apnea. It is a home sleep test that measures five channels of sleep data, including airflow, oximetry, heart rate, respiratory effort, and sound. Patients sleep in the comfort of their homes during the test. Their data is then analyzed by their team, and recommendations are made.

If you happen to live at a high altitude or have chronic obstructive pulmonary disease (COPD) or chronic bronchitis, you might not be getting enough oxygen during the day. Use your pulse oximeter to test your oxygen levels several times as you go about your day. You may need to use a CPAP machine at night, and during the day you may need to find other ways to boost your oxygen levels, including exercise with oxygen therapy (EWOT).[3]

For some of my sleep apnea patients, eliminating dairy (especially cheese) dramatically improved their symptoms.

Your Brain Needs Its Sleep

Getting enough sleep is near the top of the list of all the steps to prevent, slow, manage, stop, or reverse Alzheimer's and dementia. It seems insignificant, too "normal," something that we ignore all the time, but it is vital.

New research about the brain is coming out that would shock most people if they knew it.

Alzheimer's and dementia patients always have amyloid plaque buildup in the hippocampus area of the brain. But, believe it or not, sleep is one of the most effective ways to clear out that dreaded amyloid plaque from your brain!

While you sleep, a lot is happening in your brain:

- **Processing data:** The facts and experiences of your day need to be processed before they can be cataloged and stored. This process happens during restorative sleep.[4] Then your processing centers are ready for a new day.

- **Proper storage:** Sleep consolidates memories and helps your brain categorize short-term memories into long-term memories, declutter unnecessary bits of information, and store memories properly.[5] That means your memories are right where you put them, which directly helps with short-term and long-term memory.

- **Self-cleaning:** The brain's waste disposal system (the glymphatic system, similar to the lymphatic system) sweeps out old cells and removes toxic debris, including amyloid plaque.[6] This cleanup of your brain, especially your hippocampus, directly decreases your risk of Alzheimer's and dementia.

While the brain is in its incredibly efficient self-cleaning mode, the deeper you sleep, the better. Deep sleep speeds up the removal of the amyloid plaque by ten to twenty times! Interestingly, sleeping on your side has been found to clear the most amyloid plaque from the brain.

Lack of sleep does just the opposite and decreases your focus, memory, learning, and other skills.[7] And as you now know, lack of sleep also increases the risk of Alzheimer's and dementia by failing to remove the amyloid plaque that builds up over time.

Simply put, get your seven to eight hours of sleep each night!

Tips for Better Sleep

A lot of people struggle with sleeping at night. According to the American Sleep Association, 30 percent of the US population have a sleeping problem, and 10 percent have chronic insomnia.[8]

No matter how you count it, that's tens of millions of people every night. If you don't want to be part of that number, here are my top tips for getting a good night's sleep:

1. Stick to a schedule. My brain struggled a lot when I worked all night on call. If your work isn't keeping you up, simply decide when you want to go to bed and when you want to get up. Then set that schedule in cement (as much as you can). I go to bed at 10 p.m. and wake up at 6 a.m., and I keep it consistent, even on weekends. Get seven to eight hours of sleep consistently. It is both getting the necessary amount of sleep as well as being consistent that provide health benefits.

2. Make sure your bedroom is dark. Light increases your cortisol production and interferes with your melatonin production. Your body makes melatonin when it's dark, so keeping the lights on is the reverse of what your body needs.

3. Keep it cool. I recommend that your bedroom be at least 69–70 degrees. That temperature seems to work best for most people.

4. Use white noise. White noise is background noise that drowns out distracting sounds that would keep you up or wake you up at night. I have a white noise machine in my bedroom but not beside my bed. There are also white noise apps for your phone and white noise videos on YouTube with completely black screens that will play for hours while you sleep.

5. Cover small lights. Turn your alarm clock sideways so the red letters aren't staring at you all night. I cover the small light on my white noise machine with black tape. If you have blinking lights anywhere in your bedroom, cover them or reposition them.

6. Don't exercise right before bed. Exercise boosts your cortisol and adrenaline levels, which keep you awake. So if you plan to exercise in the evenings, make sure you are finished at least three hours before bedtime.

7. Eat your starches at dinner. Of course, you don't have to eat starch at dinner, but if you are going to eat starch, I find dinner is the best time. It makes me drowsy, and I'd rather be drowsy at night than during the day.

8. Consider using blue-blocking glasses. This may be especially helpful if you watch TV or work late at night. Some recommend using blue-blocking glasses within the last three hours before bed. I prefer instead to dim my lights at night. But if blue-blocking glasses help you, then certainly do it.

9. Minimize electromagnetic field (EMF). This often includes computers, Wi-Fi, alarm systems, cell phones, and more and can really affect some people's sleep.[9] I recommend putting all electronic devices at least six feet from your bed at night.

10. Consider aromatherapy. Many patients have had great success with essential oils, such as lavender oil, at night. It helps to relax their muscles and promote sleep. If it helps you, do it.

11. Consider a weighted blanket. Many people swear by their weighted blankets. For some, it helps them sleep.

12. Consider a special pillow and mattress. Many pillows and mattresses out there promise a good night's sleep. This is totally up to you, but if you find the secret pillow that helps you sleep, make it part of your daily routine. Get a comfortable mattress. Remember, your bed is your most important piece of furniture since you spend about 33 percent of your life in it.

What about sleeping supplements?

That's a good question. For the most part, I don't recommend prescription sleeping pills for people traveling and (for only a few days) trying to cope with the differences between time zones. Melatonin is a great supplement for these patients.

Prescription sleeping pills are not for long-term use. I can't tell you how many people I have met who are fully addicted to their sleeping pills.

Healthy natural supplements that help you sleep are a different thing entirely. I may have a patient combine two or more of these supplements since they work by different mechanisms.

I often recommend the following:

- magnesium threonate: 2,000 milligrams at bedtime, which contains only 144 milligrams of elemental magnesium. Magnesium's sedative properties increase your melatonin, decrease your circulating cortisol, and increase your sleep quality. Studies have found magnesium threonate to improve memory in older adults.[10]

- melatonin: 1–10 milligrams for adults, about an hour before bed and again in the middle of the night (if needed). Start low and go slow. I take 10 milligrams at bedtime and 10 milligrams more if I awaken during the night. But some patients need more.

- GABA. Most people are low in GABA (gamma-aminobutyric acid), a neurotransmitter that has a calming effect on your body and helps one fall asleep. I recommend GABA 500–700 milligrams, one to two capsules at bedtime for women and men.

- 5HTP (5 hydroxytryptophan): This amino acid converts to serotonin and helps you sleep. I usually recommend 150–200 milligrams at bedtime. (Do not take with SSRI meds such as Prozac.)

- bioidentical micronized progesterone: Some women need this. I recommend 100–150 milligrams about an hour before bed, and some women need more.

For more information on natural sleep supplements, please refer to *The New Bible Cure for Sleep Disorders.*

Ideally, you can train your body to go to sleep and sleep deeply without any supplements simply by winding down before bedtime, reading the Bible, or listening to calming music. But if you need supplements, start with one and add others if needed. Start low and go slow. I normally like listening to relaxing music by Tim Janis (on YouTube) before bed.

I recommend that you try these tips every night for the next month. If your sleep has improved even a little bit, keep going.

Sleep is vital, but it is easily disturbed. Calmly but consistently work to improve your sleep.

KEY 2: MANAGE YOUR STRESS

Stress is one of those things in life that is good for your body and brain, but only in small amounts. Temporary stress makes you sharp and gives you energy. Like caffeine, it helps you focus on whatever is required of you. Mild to moderate short-term stress enhances memory.[11]

However, chronic, long-term stress has the opposite effect. When stress becomes severe, memory declines.[12]

This unrelenting type of stress is often found in people with anxiety, depression, chronic illness, PTSD, and chronic pain. I've even seen chronic stress be caused by worry, stressful jobs, bad marriages, family dynamics (sick child, child on drugs, family member in jail), the commute to work, and harmful routines.

Long-term stress is harmful to your body in many areas, causing

- belly fat,
- elevated blood sugar levels,
- higher cholesterol levels,
- hormone deficiencies,
- hormone imbalances,
- increased blood pressure,
- increased cortisol levels,
- increased risk for disease,
- weakened immune system, and
- weight gain.

But regarding your brain, long-term stress is literally like poison, bringing with it

- an increased risk of cognitive issues,[13]
- decreased memory performance,[14]
- hippocampus shrinkage,[15]
- death of neurons in the hippocampus,
- inhibited glucose absorption (primarily in the hippocampus, where it's sorely needed), and
- damaged hippocampus function: forgetting, depression, memory loss, and more.[16]

Chronic stress keeps your body and brain in a heightened state of unrest. It's like being "on" or in emergency mode all the time. The body and brain simply can't handle the pressure over time.

Stress is such an important issue that I wrote an entire book on the subject (*Stress Less*). Many years later I still think stress is one of the biggest silent killers today. Disease is almost always present in those with chronic stress, and with so much stress out there, it's little wonder why disease is so rampant.

How to Handle Stress

My advice for those under chronic stress is always the same: learn to cope with your stress, manage your stress, avoid more stress, and remove your stress.

Yes, it's easier said than done, but doing nothing is not an answer either. Though some stress is unavoidable, you would be surprised at how many people just keep going, not evaluating or changing anything in their daily routines. That's not wise or healthy.

Truly, if you want different results, you must do something different. That applies to all areas of your health.

My recommendations for dealing with stress and maintaining your health are a mix of several practical options that have worked with many patients over the years:

- Do deep breathing exercises.
- Drink green tea without sugar. (It contains L-theanine, which is calming.)
- Exercise.
- Foster an attitude of gratitude: journal ten things you are grateful for every day.
- Get counseling if you need it.
- Get more sleep.
- Go out on a date.
- Have fun doing things you enjoy.
- Laugh every day. (Get at least ten belly laughs a day.)
- Listen to motivating podcasts.
- Listen to praise-and-worship music.
- Listen to relaxing music (such as Tim Janis on YouTube—my favorite is "Beautiful Sunrise").
- Meditate on God's Word.
- Play with your grandkids.
- Pray.

- Read or listen to good books.
- Read the Bible.
- Say no to more demands placed on you.
- Slow your day's hectic pace.
- Take a break.
- Turn off the news.
- Use essential oils.
- Walk your pet.
- Watch good clean comedy.

The truth of Proverbs 17:22 is amazingly accurate: "A merry heart does good like a medicine, but a broken spirit dries the bones."

All these recommendations may seem like insignificant little steps, but each is a step forward, which counts when it comes to lowering stress levels.

Every effort to handle stress is done on purpose. You must choose it and make it happen. Seldom will it simply happen by itself. With stress, it is usually necessary to be proactive.

You are not a "human doing" but a "human being." Stop the excessive doing and just be still. Be still and know God!

As always, getting to the root of the problem and fixing whatever is causing stress to your body and brain is the best answer. It may take you time to do so, but you must do it.

For most people, their stressful lives are of their own making. Their stress is self-generated.[17]

But stress on your body and brain is simply not something you want to live with any longer. Your memory depends on you minimizing and coping with stress. Jesus said it best in John 16:33: "I have told you all this so that you may have peace in me. Here on earth you will have many trials and sorrows. But take heart, because I have overcome the world" (NLT).

KEY 3: MAKE EXERCISE A HABIT

When I cut back on my day's busy schedule determined to make room for exercise, I set myself up for success by viewing that half to one hour as a scheduled appointment I have to keep. Maybe write it on your calendar as your "doctor's appointment," because you certainly don't want to miss those.

However you choose to do it, don't miss your exercise window. Your body and brain need exercise in a very big way.

Unfortunately, most people don't stick to their exercise routines if they even have one to begin with. Statistics show that 80 percent of the US population doesn't get enough exercise.[18] I would expect the same numbers globally because we are all creatures of habit.

IT'S A FACT

Exercise is the single most important strategy to prevent and improve memory loss.[19]

As you would expect, those who need to exercise the most are not getting it. According to the CDC, more than 65 percent of the younger, fitter population (ages eighteen to twenty-four) get enough exercise, and then it's all downhill from there. Of those over sixty-five, around 40 percent are getting the exercise they need, and of those over seventy-five, around 32 percent are exercising adequately.[20]

The older population, which is right in the peak ages for Alzheimer's and dementia and countless sicknesses and diseases, is not getting the exercise their bodies and brains so desperately need.

Everyone knows exercise is good. That's not a question. Some even argue that the best preventive measure against getting Alzheimer's or dementia is exercise. Others say that simply being active is the best defense against cognitive decline. Clearly, exercise of any sort is good for your body and brain.

What Counts as Exercise?

Patients always have questions about exercise: "How much do I need to do? What is the best exercise for protecting the brain? What are my options? How much time do I need to exercise? Do I need to join a gym? What will this cost me?"

Some are asking for their family and friends. I've had many ask what exercises or exercise routines their parents should be doing to fight back against Alzheimer's or dementia.

If you are trying to prevent, slow, manage, stop, or reverse Alzheimer's or dementia, then I suggest the following exercise routine.

Your Healthy Brain Exercise Routine

1. Start low.

Start where you are and with what you have. Walking is a good option; you don't need a gym membership, you can work it around your schedule, and you can do it with your spouse or friends.

- Light exercise: twenty minutes, three times per week

- Medium-light exercise: twenty to thirty minutes, three to five times per week

It may not be as aerobic or muscle strengthening as other forms of exercise, but walking is good and certainly counts as being active. Using a treadmill works just as well.

This routine will probably get you three thousand steps (about 1.3–1.5 miles) in a day, which usually takes about twenty minutes, and though this is not intensive exercise, it is still enough to benefit and protect your brain. You may want to track your progress with a pedometer or Fitbit.

If you have a dog, this is a great excuse to go for a walk, and it makes exercise an easy habit to maintain. You may want to consider getting a dog not only for the fun and companionship, but for the exercise benefits you will receive.

2. Increase slowly.

Maintain your walking but begin to add both aerobic and strengthening exercises as well. Both are known to be good for a healthy, fit brain.[21] For aerobic exercise, you may want to ride a bike in a park, swim laps in a pool, ride a stationary or recumbent bike, use an elliptical or a rowing machine, or engage in one of many other effective exercise options.

Light to moderate weight training that tones and builds muscles is good to incorporate. That might mean using free weights or a machine (at home or the gym); either will do the job.

The goal at this stage is to increase—to move from walking to additional forms of exercise that burn more calories, build muscle, and benefit your body and brain to a greater degree. This would be about thirty to forty-five minutes a day, four to five times per week.

When this has become a habit, it's time to consider taking it up another notch.

3. Build up.

At this level, you may be walking four or five times a week (perhaps by walking your dog), getting your aerobic exercise in by whatever method you prefer, but now it's time to increase your overall exercise routine to about sixty minutes a day, five to six days a week.

Of the many options, you want to be sure to include a good portion of weight training (at home or the gym), because adding muscle is a multiplier to all your efforts. For example, weight training speeds up any weight loss efforts (even stationary muscles are burning energy), expedites the removal of amyloid plaque from the brain, and exponentially decreases cognitive decline.

IT'S A FACT

Following any four of these five (according to Cardiff University) may reduce your risk of dementia by 60 percent:

1. regular exercise

2. *not smoking*

3. *acceptable body mass index (BMI)*

4. *high fruit and vegetable intake*

5. *low/moderate alcohol intake*[22]

We are not talking about bodybuilding! This is still strength training, small-scale muscle building, and it's giving your body what it needs at a level you can easily maintain.

Adding a little muscle will help prevent sarcopenia (muscle loss usually due to aging), brain atrophy, and cognitive impairment.[23]

4. Go high.

With brain health and reducing the risk of Alzheimer's and dementia, you can take the approach that more is almost always better. That does not mean you need to be discouraged or feel pressured to run triathlons or marathons. Not at all. It simply means that the more you can do, the better it is for your body and brain.

If you are physically and aerobically fit but want to increase your physical activity, then I suggest high-intensity interval training (HIIT).

For me, this is just twelve to fifteen minutes a day, five to six days a week. I ride a recumbent bike for a couple of minutes, then spend one minute max pedaling at max resistance. This gets my heart rate up to around 145–155. Then I back it off to half the resistance for one minute, and my heart rate slows to around 125–135. Then I spend one minute max pedaling at max resistance. My heart rate goes back up.

Back and forth, I do this for about twelve to fifteen minutes, finishing it off with a couple of minutes at less resistance to cool down.

HIIT works the body, heart, lungs, muscles, and more and is especially effective in helping to strengthen your brain.

There are many different ways to create your HIIT workout. Maybe you prefer running, riding a bike outside, riding a stationary or recumbent bike, using a ski machine or elliptical machine, or some other exercise—that's up to you. I prefer the recumbent bike because it is less pressure on my knees, but you do what you like best and what will most easily become a habit.

Aim for four to eight high-intensity periods and the same number of slow periods, with a two-minute warm-up to start and a two-minute cooldown to end.

You do need to know your maximum heart rate. Take 220 and subtract your age. Use that number as your max heart rate. With HIIT, you want to hit 90–100 percent of your max heart rate four to eight times.

For HIIT you need to be healthy and not have heart disease. It's fast, and you get the benefits in about fifteen minutes. The American College of Sports Medicine and the American Heart Association recommend exercise testing for those at moderate risk of heart disease. They do not recommend stress testing in men less than forty-five years and women less than fifty-five years unless one or more coronary risk factors are present (other than age or gender).[24] Coronary risk factors include (1) high LDL cholesterol, (2) low HDL cholesterol, (3) high blood pressure, (4) family history of heart disease, (5) diabetes, (6) smoking, (7) being postmenopausal, for women, and (8) being older than forty-five, for men.[25]

IT'S A FACT

Cognitive decline can be avoided with simple everyday exercises, a new study suggests.[26]

EXERCISE MULTIPLIES YOUR EFFORTS

Exercise is unique because its benefits reach every part of your body down to the cellular level. But what's more, exercise seems to pull all the parts together.

For instance, your efforts to break free of insulin resistance are far more effective when you add exercise. The same goes for removing toxins, intermittent fasting, getting a good night's sleep, managing your stress, and more. If I were to put a number on it, I would estimate that exercise is a five to ten times multiplier of the effectiveness of any action to decrease the risk of Alzheimer's and dementia.

Exercise is beneficial to good health and helps with memory loss. You can't go wrong with adding more exercise to your day.

YOUR EXERCISE HABIT

If you have a medical condition, you may want to consult your doctor first. Usually, starting low and going slow is safe for most people. It's also good practice and one of the easiest ways to establish a habit.

When it comes right down to it, when you have made exercise a habit, you are well on your way to reducing your risk of Alzheimer's and dementia.

Interestingly, making exercise a habit is a mental game. It requires effort and several weeks to establish a habit. You would think your brain, which benefits from exercise, would be quicker to accept and set the habit!

IT'S A FACT

To calculate your maximum heart rate: subtract your age from 220. Moderate exercise will be about 70 percent of that, and higher intensity exercise will be 90–100 percent.

Unfortunately, it doesn't work that way. It requires effort to start and keep a habit, but this is your health and longevity we are talking about, so you have more than enough reason to press forward.

If you, like me, have one copy of the ApoE4 gene that increases the risk of Alzheimer's and dementia, then you have an extra reason to keep up the exercise habit. If you have two copies of the ApoE4 gene, exercise needs to be part of your daily routine.

Never forget, as I've said many times, no matter what your genes might be, the biggest factors determining your health and longevity are the choices you make (exercise, diet, sleep, stress, attitude, and more). Having an ApoE4 gene is no guarantee of anything.

It's never too late to start. Research has found a similarly lower mortality risk between those who have exercised all their lives and those who started in middle age (forty to sixty-one).[27] The point is you can (if you haven't already) start now and enjoy the benefits of exercise. Your body and brain will love you for it!

YOUR TO-DO LIST FOR A HEALTHY BRAIN

❑ Avoid heavy metals (use chelation agents to remove them from your body).

❑ Avoid mercury (in silver fillings, certain fish, certain cosmetics).

❑ Avoid arsenic (in some drinking water and food).

❑ Avoid lead (in water, gasoline, paint, cigarette smoke, pipes, toys, city dust).

❑ Avoid cadmium (in excessive amounts of chocolate, smoking, tobacco).

❑ Test to see if you are part of the 25 percent of the population that is sensitive to mold. (See appendix B.)

❑ Treat your body and home for mold (if needed).

❑ Avoid certain antihistamines long-term (Benadryl and Atarax).

❑ Avoid certain anticholinergic medications long-term. (Fix the problem; medications are bandages.)

❑ Avoid too much copper. (Take zinc supplements to maintain a 1-to-1 ratio.)

❑ Avoid artificial sweeteners, especially aspartame. (Minimize sugar intake as well.)

❑ Decrease alcohol intake. (Dry red wine, in small amounts, may be OK.)

❑ Stop drinking alcohol if you have the ApoE4 gene. (Any amount of alcohol increases the risk of Alzheimer's and dementia for those with the ApoE4 gene.[28])

❑ Avoid trans fats (often in processed food).

❏ Avoid unnecessary anesthesia. (Local anesthesia is OK; keep oxygen levels high, and take glutathione supplement after surgery to clear it out of your body. See appendix B.)

❏ Avoid marijuana.

❏ Eradicate any chronic infections (cold sores, gingivitis, periodontal disease, chronic sinusitis, chronic bronchitis, chronic viral diseases, chronic Lyme disease, and Lyme disease coinfections).

❏ Correct insulin resistance (lose weight, reverse prediabetes and type 2 diabetes).

❏ Quench inflammation. (Fix it; don't patch it.)

❏ Restore your leaky gut.

❏ Do intermittent fasting regularly.

❏ Consistently get a good night's sleep.

❏ Manage your stress. (Remove stressors if you can.)

❏ Create an exercise habit (and stick to it).

❏ Balance your hormones. (Optimize if need be.)

❏ Feed your body the right food (a healthy keto diet or a healthy Mediterranean-keto diet).

❏ Fuel your brain daily.

❏ Strengthen your brain. (Every single day, exercise your brain.)

❏ Get ten belly laughs a day.

CONCLUSION

THE BEST OF YOUR LIFE FOR THE REST OF YOUR LIFE

A S WE COME to the end of this transformative journey through *Health Zone Essentials*, I want to express my deepest gratitude for allowing me to be your guide on this path toward holistic health. The journey we've embarked upon is not just a fleeting one—it's a lifelong commitment to nurturing your body, mind, and spirit. The title of this conclusion, "The Best of Your Life for the Rest of Your Life," encapsulates the essence of the journey you've undertaken and the boundless potential that lies ahead.

Throughout these pages we've explored the intricacies of gut health, the nourishing power of the Mediterranean-keto diet, the revitalizing effects of intermittent fasting, the harmony of balanced hormones, and how to safeguard our brain health. Each part has provided you with insights, practices, and knowledge that contribute to the symphony of wellness that is your life.

Now, using the knowledge from these chapters, it's time to weave your own wellness tapestry. You have the tools to create a personalized plan that encompasses all the aspects of health we've discussed. Remember, this isn't about perfection; it's about progress. It's about consistently making choices that honor your well-being and reflect your commitment to vibrant living.

As you move forward, I encourage you to embrace wellness as a lifestyle, not a temporary endeavor. Allow the wisdom you've gained to infuse your daily routines, your choices at the dinner table, and your mindset as you navigate challenges. Let self-care become second nature, and remember that small, consistent steps lead to remarkable transformations.

When you invest in your health, you're investing in a future filled with vitality, energy, and joy. You're laying the foundation for a life where you can truly be the best version of yourself—not just for a short period, but for the rest of your life. It's a future where you can savor the moments, embrace new challenges, and cherish the gift of a life well-lived.

As I reflect on the words I've shared here and envision how you will be transformed, I'm filled with gratitude—for your commitment to your health, your openness to new ideas, and your trust in my guidance. Remember that this journey is ongoing; it's not a destination but a continuous evolution.

In times of uncertainty, stress, or doubt, I invite you to return to the protocols outlined in these pages. Draw strength from the practices you've learned, the wisdom you've acquired, and the understanding that you have the power to shape your own health story.

Thank you for walking this path with me. Thank you for valuing your well-being and recognizing the importance of a holistic approach to health. Remember that you are not alone on this journey. Let the knowledge you've gained serve as a lifelong companion.

As you close this book and step back into your world, I urge you to stand strong in your commitment to holistic health. Be mindful of the choices you make. And let the lessons learned guide you to a future filled with health, vitality, and the joy of living fully.

APPENDIX A

RECIPES FOR OPTIMAL WELLNESS

T HIS APPENDIX OFFERS tasty recipes that follow the progression of parts 1 and 2 of *Dr. Colbert's Health Zone Essentials*. First you'll discover recipes that help you restore your GI tract and lay the foundation for your overall health. Then you'll find Mediterranean-keto recipes that define your healthy eating lifestyle going forward.

RECIPES THAT RESTORE GUT HEALTH

Smoothie

8 ounces almond or low-fat, low-sugar coconut milk
2 tablespoons avocado oil
½–1 scoop egg white protein (if not sensitive to egg) or collagen protein (see appendix B)
¼ cup frozen berries
Stevia

Blend first four ingredients. Sweeten to taste with stevia. Add ice if desired.

Chocolate Smoothie

½ teaspoon dark sugar-free cocoa
½ teaspoon stevia
1 tablespoon almond butter
1 tablespoon avocado oil
1 scoop chocolate hydrolyzed collagen protein
8 ounces almond or low-fat, low-sugar coconut milk

Blend all ingredients. Add ice if desired.

Healthy Gut Zone Flapjacks

2 eggs
½ cup green banana flour or sweet potato flour
Pinch of salt
Water
Pinch of cinnamon
Fresh blueberries or blackberries
Avocado oil
Grass-fed butter

Combine eggs, flour, salt, water, and cinnamon. Pour into a griddle or frying pan; flip to brown both sides. Simmer berries in 2 tablespoons avocado oil over low heat. Top flapjacks with berries and a pat of grass-fed butter.

Grilled Chicken Salad

Large salad greens
Onions, chopped or sliced
Mushrooms, chopped or sliced
Celery, chopped or sliced
Fresh parsley
2–4 tablespoons dressing made with avocado oil such as
    Primal Kitchen's (may add lemon juice and/or vinegar)
3–6 ounces boneless organic free-range chicken breast,
    grilled
Grilled onions

Toss salad greens with vegetables and parsley. Drizzle with olive oil, and top with grilled chicken and grilled onions.

Curry Soup

Gut-friendly veggies of your choice (such as onions, carrots,
    celery, garlic, broccoli, mushrooms), diced or chopped
1 boneless organic free-range chicken breast, diced or shred-
    ded
1 tablespoon yellow curry powder
2 cups organic chicken stock
½ cup low-fat coconut milk
1 tablespoon freshly squeezed lime juice

4–6 tablespoons extra-virgin olive oil or avocado oil
Salt

In a stockpot, combine your choice of gut-friendly veggies with chicken breast, curry powder, chicken stock, coconut milk, and lime juice. Season with salt as desired. Simmer for 25 minutes on medium heat. After simmering and before serving, add olive oil or avocado oil. Serves 2.

Grilled Salmon Salad

Romaine lettuce, chopped
Onions, chopped or sliced
Mushrooms, chopped or sliced
Carrots, chopped or sliced
Celery, chopped or sliced
2–4 tablespoons extra-virgin olive oil (may add lemon juice
and/or vinegar)
3–6 ounces wild salmon, grilled

Toss romaine lettuce with vegetables. Drizzle with olive oil, and top with grilled salmon.

Tortilla-less Chicken Soup

1 small onion, diced
1–2 teaspoons minced garlic
3 cups organic chicken stock
9–12 ounces boneless organic free-range chicken breast,
boiled and shredded
1 tablespoon freshly squeezed lime juice
⅓–½ cup fresh cilantro leaves, chopped
1 avocado, sliced or cubed
½–1 cup mushrooms (if desired)
½–1 cup broccoli (if desired)
6–8 tablespoons extra-virgin olive oil

In a stockpot, combine first nine ingredients. Simmer 25 minutes on medium heat. After simmering and before serving, add olive oil. Serves 3.

Millet Bread French Toast

2 large brown organic pastured eggs
1 teaspoon organic vanilla extract
½ teaspoon ground cinnamon
½ cup low-fat coconut milk
Stevia to taste
2 slices millet bread
Avocado oil
¼ cup berries (if desired)
Grass-fed butter (if desired)

Make a batter by whisking together eggs, vanilla extract, cinnamon, coconut milk, and stevia. Soak each slice of millet bread in batter. Cook in skillet using avocado oil over low heat. Add berries simmered in 2 tablespoons avocado oil and a pat of grass-fed butter as a topping if desired. Serves 2.

Simple Turkey Salad

Spinach
2–4 tablespoons olive oil (may add lemon juice and/or vinegar)
3–6 ounces turkey
Green mango and/or green papaya, sliced

Toss spinach with olive oil. Top with turkey and add slices of green mango and/or green papaya.

Chicken Salad

1 boneless organic free-range chicken breast
2 celery stalks
½ onion
Salt
Pepper
½ cup pecans
⅓ cup avocado oil mayonnaise
1 tablespoon fresh dill, chopped (if desired)
1 tablespoon Dijon mustard (if desired)
2 tablespoons extra-virgin olive oil or avocado oil
2 large romaine lettuce leaves

Boil chicken breast in water with celery stalks, onion, salt, and pepper for 20–25 minutes. Once cooked, chill chicken in refrigerator while making rest of salad. Chop the cooked celery and onion into small pieces. Add pecans, mayonnaise, and, if desired, fresh dill and Dijon mustard. Season with salt and pepper to taste. Add shredded chicken and olive oil or avocado oil to rest of ingredients. Mix well. Serve 1–2 scoops on large leaf of romaine lettuce. Serves 2.

Optional: You may make a sandwich using millet bread. However, a low-carb diet works better for the first month.

Grass-Fed Beef Soup

> 2–4 cups organic beef stock
> Gut-friendly veggies of your choice (such as onions, carrots, mushrooms, and broccoli), diced or chopped
> Garlic
> 8 ounces grass-fed, grass-finished lean filet mignon, grilled and diced
> Salt
> Pepper
> 4–6 tablespoons extra-virgin olive oil or avocado oil

In a stockpot, combine first four ingredients. Season with salt and pepper to taste. Simmer for 25 minutes or longer. After simmering and before serving, add olive oil or avocado oil. Serves 2.

Wild Shrimp Gumbo

> 8 ounces wild shrimp
> 2–3 cups organic chicken stock
> ½ cup onion, chopped
> ½ cup celery, chopped
> 2 garlic cloves, minced
> ½ cup fresh okra
> Salt
> Pepper
> 4–6 tablespoons extra-virgin olive oil

In a stockpot, combine first six ingredients. Add salt and pepper to taste. Simmer for 25–30 minutes. After simmering and before serving, add olive oil. Serves 2.

Tongol Tuna Salad

1 can tongol tuna
2 celery stalks
½ onion
½ cup pecans
⅓ cup avocado oil mayonnaise
1 tablespoon fresh dill, chopped (if desired)
1 tablespoon Dijon mustard (if desired)
Salt
Pepper
2 tablespoons extra-virgin olive oil or avocado oil
Green mango, sliced
2 large romaine lettuce leaves

Open can of tongol tuna, and chill tuna in refrigerator while making rest of salad. Chop celery and onion into small pieces. Add pecans, mayonnaise, and, if desired, fresh dill and Dijon mustard. Season with salt and pepper to taste. Add tuna and olive oil or avocado oil to rest of ingredients. Add slices of green mango. Mix well. Serve 1–2 scoops on large leaf of romaine lettuce. Serves 2.

Optional: You may make a tuna sandwich using millet bread.

Bone Broth Soup

BONE BROTH:

2 quarts water
2 pounds pastured animal bones (chicken, beef, or a mix)
¼ pound onion (or ½ large onion)
2 cloves garlic
1 tablespoon vinegar
1 teaspoon salt or more to taste
½ teaspoon black pepper or to taste

Combine ingredients and slowcook for 24 to 48 hours or pressure-cook for 4 hours. Makes 5 to 6 cups.

SOUP:

2 cups bone broth
Cooked boneless, skinless chicken OR grass-fed, grass-finished low-fat beef or steak, shredded or cubed
½ cup onions, chopped

½ cup broccoli, chopped
½ cup celery, chopped
2 garlic cloves, minced
Salt
Pepper
4–6 tablespoons extra-virgin olive oil or avocado oil

In a stockpot, combine first six ingredients. Season with salt and pepper to taste. Simmer for 25 minutes. After simmering and before serving, add olive oil or avocado oil. Serves 2.

Kale and Veggie Salad With Chicken

4 cups (packed) kale leaves, torn, with stems removed
½ cup avocado, chopped
⅓ cup red onion
½ cup English cucumber, deseeded and chopped
Handful of pomegranate seeds
1 radish, thinly sliced
1 celery stalk, chopped
2–4 tablespoons extra-virgin olive oil
2 tablespoons freshly squeezed lime juice
¼ cup cilantro, chopped (if desired)
3–6 ounces boneless organic free-range chicken, grilled

Toss together first ten ingredients. Top with sliced-up grilled chicken.

Spicy Ginger Salad With Chicken or Beef

Cabbage (green, purple, or mixed), chopped or shredded
Carrots, chopped or sliced
Radishes, sliced
Parsnips, chopped or sliced
Onions, chopped or sliced
Celery, chopped or sliced
2 tablespoons fresh ginger
2–4 tablespoons extra-virgin olive oil (may add lemon juice and/or vinegar)
3–6 ounces lean grass-fed, grass-finished beef OR boneless organic free-range chicken, grilled and cut in strips

Toss cabbage with other veggies. Grate or dice ginger over top. Drizzle with olive oil, and top with strips of grilled beef or chicken.

Creamy Carrot Chicken and Coconut Soup

> 2–3 large carrots, finely chopped
> 14-ounce can low-fat coconut milk
> 1 onion, finely chopped
> 1 tablespoon curry powder
> 1 teaspoon fresh ginger, minced
> 2 cups organic vegetable or chicken broth
> 8 ounces boneless organic free-range chicken, boiled and
>   shredded
> Salt
> Pepper
> 4–6 tablespoons extra-virgin olive oil or avocado oil

In a stockpot, combine first seven ingredients. Season with salt and pepper to taste. Simmer for 25 minutes. After simmering and before serving, add olive oil or avocado oil. Serves 2.

Tasty Mediterranean-Keto Meal Ideas and Recipes

The Mediterranean-keto lifestyle enables you to keep off weight and avoid sickness and disease. These benefits can be the foundation of a healthy lifestyle that you get to enjoy for the rest of your life. The core of this lifestyle is healthy fats (e.g., olive oil, avocado oil, nut oils), fruits, a lot of non-starchy vegetables, small to moderate amounts of legumes, nuts, moderate amounts of lean meats and fish, and occasional wine, but this lifestyle is still low in sugars and carbs.

The Mediterranean-keto recipes in the following meal plan incorporate more carbs than a strictly keto diet and follow these macro levels: 50–55 percent fats, 20–25 percent proteins, and 20–25 percent carbs. Many people find 75–100 grams of net carbs to be their sweet spot for maintenance. Keep in mind that higher-carb food such as brown rice, gluten-free pasta, sweet potatoes, and cassava should only be occasional food a few times a week, though a serving of legumes each day is OK. As I mentioned previously, it's best to use dry legumes, soak them overnight, and pressure-cook them to remove inflammatory lectins. Then add them to a recipe or as a side.

If you want or need to go through a keto diet for weight loss before switching to the more relaxed Mediterranean-keto lifestyle, look for the "strictly keto" modifications noted with some recipes. To lose weight, women shouldn't exceed 1,600 calories per day and men shouldn't exceed 2,000 to 2,400 calories per day. That amounts to roughly 450 to 600 calories per meal for women and 600 to 800 calories per meal for men. Men can increase their portions or add more oil to their meals to increase their caloric intake.

Again, remember your macros. Keep your net carbs at 20 grams a day to stay in ketosis (fat-burning mode), and aim for 75 percent fats, 5 percent carbs, and 20 percent proteins.

For women at 1,600 calories eating three meals per day, that means approximately

- 44 grams of fats per meal (around 3.33 tablespoons of fats per meal),
- 27 grams of proteins per meal (around 4 ounces of proteins per meal), and
- 7 grams of carbs per meal.

For men at 2,400 calories eating three meals per day, that means approximately

- 67 grams of fats per meal (around 5 tablespoons of fats per meal),
- 40 grams of proteins per meal (around 6 ounces of proteins per meal), and
- 10 grams of carbs per meal (or 7 grams per meal if you choose 20 grams of carbs per day).

If you are starting at a different number of calories per day, divide your daily calorie goal by your intended number of meals per day, and keep each meal within that range. As usual on a keto diet, watch the carbs from fruits, higher-carb nuts and vegetables, starches, and beans.

193

As I mentioned, I have found that after their bodies get used to being in ketosis, many people can increase their net carbs to around 50–75 grams per day and will still be in ketosis—some can go as high as 100 grams per day.

If your starting point is the Mediterranean-keto lifestyle, then 50 grams of carbs per day is recommended to begin as your body gets used to burning fat instead of sugar for fuel. Then you can slowly increase to 75–100 grams of carbs per day. Some can go as high as 125 grams of carbs per day and maintain a healthy weight. If you find yourself gaining weight, reduce the amount of carbs you're eating each day.

Mix and match the following meal ideas until you get familiar with the types and amounts of food to eat on a daily basis. Then, after you have practiced with these recipes for a few weeks, seek out other recipes or experiment with your own. I believe you'll find, as I did, that a Mediterranean-keto diet isn't just healthy; it's delicious.

BREAKFASTS

Breakfast Scramble

> 1 teaspoon grass-fed ghee
> 3 tablespoons avocado oil, divided
> ½ cup yams, diced
> ¼ cup broccoli, chopped
> ¼ cup onions, chopped
> ¼ cup button mushrooms, sliced
> ¼ cup spinach, shredded
> 2 organic pasture-raised eggs
> 1 link cooked chicken sausage or 2–3 slices of turkey or
>   regular bacon (nitrate/nitrite-free), diced
> ¼ cup berries

Heat ghee and 1 tablespoon of avocado oil over medium heat. Add the yams. Cook 3–4 minutes. Add veggies and cook 3–4 minutes more, until tender. In a small bowl, whisk eggs. Add to veggies and stir until desired doneness. Top with diced meat of your choice. Drizzle with remaining avocado oil. Serve with a side of berries. (1 serving)

Mediterranean-keto:

Calories: 567; net carbs: 27 grams

Strictly keto: Women use 2 eggs, men use 3 eggs, and omit the yams and berries.

Calories (2 eggs): 458; net carbs: 5 grams

Calories (3 eggs): 529; net carbs: 5 grams

Fruit and Almond Pancakes

FRUIT SYRUP:

½ cup strawberries
½ cup chopped peaches
2 ½ tablespoons avocado oil
1 ½ tablespoons grass-fed ghee
½ teaspoon debittered stevia (optional)

PANCAKES:

4 large eggs
½ cup almond flour
1 tablespoon stevia (debittered)
¼ teaspoon baking powder
¼ cup avocado oil
¼ cup sliced or slivered almonds
Coconut cream (optional)
Organic natural almond or peanut butter (optional)

Cook strawberries, peaches, 2 ½ tablespoons avocado oil, and ghee over low heat until fruit is soft. Stir in stevia and let cool. In a small bowl, whisk eggs. In a separate bowl, combine almond flour, stevia, and baking powder. Stir half of the remaining avocado oil into the eggs. Whisk dry ingredients into egg mixture. Use remaining avocado oil to grease a griddle or frying pan. Heat over medium-low heat. Ladle ¼ cup of batter onto pan. Sprinkle almonds on top of each pancake. Flip pancakes after 2–3 minutes, when edges are no longer moist. Top with fruit syrup. If desired, add a dollop of coconut cream sweetened with stevia (50 calories; 1 gram of net carbs per tablespoon), or spread natural almond butter (98 calories; 1 gram of net carbs per tablespoon) or peanut butter (94 calories; 2 grams of net carbs per tablespoon) on pancakes before topping with syrup. Makes 6 pancakes.

Mediterranean-keto:

Syrup—calories per tablespoon: 68; net carbs: 1.5 grams

Pancakes (each, without coconut cream or nut butter)—calories: 186; net carbs: 2 grams

Strictly keto: Omit the peaches from the syrup and use 1 cup strawberries. If you choose to top pancakes with nut butter, use almond butter instead of peanut butter. Suggested serving: 2 pancakes for women (372 calories; 4 grams net carbs) with 2 tablespoons syrup (135 calories; 2 grams net carbs) and 3 pancakes for men (558 calories; 6 grams net carbs) with 3 table-spoons syrup (203 calories; 3 grams net carbs).

Syrup—calories per tablespoon: 68; net carbs: 1 gram

Chocolate Peanut Butter Shake

1 cup unsweetened almond or coconut milk
½–1 teaspoon dark unsweetened cocoa powder
¼–½ teaspoon stevia (debittered)
1 tablespoon avocado or macadamia nut oil (2 tablespoons for men)
2 tablespoons organic peanut butter or almond butter
1 scoop Keto Zone chocolate hydrolyzed collagen protein powder
½ cup ice

Place all the ingredients in a blender and process until smooth. (1 serving)

Mediterranean-keto:

Calories: 437; net carbs: 5 grams

Men (with extra tablespoon avocado or macadamia nut oil)—calories: 557; net carbs: 5 grams

Strictly keto: Use almond butter.

Calories: 445; net carbs: 4 grams

Men (with extra tablespoon avocado or macadamia nut oil)—calories: 565; net carbs: 4 grams

Nutty Cereal

3 cups unsweetened shaved coconut
1 cup finely chopped walnuts, pecans, and almonds

1 tablespoon coconut oil, melted
1 tablespoon macadamia nut oil
1 tablespoon vanilla extract
½ teaspoon stevia (debittered)
1 tablespoon cinnamon
½ teaspoon sea salt

Preheat oven to 300 degrees. In bowl, mix coconut and nuts. In separate bowl, whisk oil, vanilla, stevia, cinnamon, and salt. Drizzle over nut mixture and stir well. Spread mixture onto lined baking sheet. Bake until lightly toasted, stirring occasionally. Remove from oven and cool. Makes 4 cups. Recommended serving: ⅔ cup for women and 1 cup for men served with an equal amount of unsweetened almond, coconut, or oat milk.

Mediterranean-keto:

2/3 cup without milk—calories: 377; net carbs: 6 grams

1 cup without milk—calories: 566; net carbs: 9 grams

Strictly keto: Serve with almond milk (30–40 calories; 1 gram net carbs per cup).

Salmon and Avocado Lettuce Wraps

2–4 butter lettuce leaves
1 avocado, cut into wedges
2–4 tomato slices
2–4 onion slices
6–8 ounces smoked salmon slices (my favorite is Biltmore wild Alaskan sockeye salmon)
Lemon wedges
Himalayan salt
White or black sesame seeds

Place tomato and onion slices in bottom of each butter lettuce leaf. Layer smoked salmon on top. Add 2 avocado wedges to each wrap and mash down slightly with a fork. Sprinkle with lemon juice, salt, and sesame seeds. Suggested portion size: 6 ounces salmon for women and 8 ounces salmon for men. (1 serving)

Mediterranean-keto:

> **8 ounces salmon**—calories: 541; net carbs: 7 grams

> **6 ounces salmon**—calories: 421; net carbs: 6 grams

Strictly keto: No modifications needed.

Keto Breakfast Porridge

> 2 tablespoons ground flaxseed
> 2 tablespoons ground chia seeds
> 2 tablespoons unsweetened shredded coconut
> 1–2 teaspoons granulated sweetener of choice (monk fruit, debittered stevia)
> ½ cup hot unsweetened oat, almond, or coconut milk
> ½–1 cup cold unsweetened oat, almond, or coconut milk
> 3 tablespoons chopped nuts (hazelnuts, walnuts, almonds, pecans)
> ¼ cup raspberries, strawberries, blueberries, or blackberries
> Dash of cinnamon or nutmeg (optional)
> Splash of vanilla extract (optional)

Combine dry ingredients in a small bowl. Add the hot liquid and stir well. It will be thick! Add the cold liquid, stirring until desired consistency, similar to oatmeal. Stir in nuts, berries, and spices. To prepare the night before, add an extra 4 tablespoons of liquid to thin mixture. Place it in fridge. (1 serving)

Mediterranean-keto:

> Calories: 458; net carbs: 6 grams

Strictly keto: Use coconut or almond milk.

Quick Berry Muffin

> 3 tablespoons almond flour
> 1 tablespoon coconut flour
> ½ teaspoon stevia (debittered)
> ¼ teaspoon baking powder
> Pinch of salt
> 1 large egg
> 1 teaspoon grass-fed ghee (melted and cooled)
> 2 tablespoons avocado oil (3 tablespoons for men)
> ¼ teaspoon vanilla extract
> 8 blueberries or raspberries

Whisk the flours, sweetener, baking powder, and salt in a large microwave-safe mug. In a separate small bowl, whisk the egg, ghee, oil, and vanilla. Mix into the dry ingredients. Gently stir in the berries. Smooth the top of the batter.

Place mug in the microwave for 1 minute 15 seconds. If the muffin is not cooked through, cook 15 seconds more. Carefully remove the hot mug from the microwave. Flip it upside down over a plate. Spread with ghee if desired. (1 serving)

Mediterranean-keto:

Calories (with 2 tablespoons avocado oil): 492; net carbs: 6 grams

Calories (with 3 tablespoons avocado oil): 612; net carbs: 6 grams

Strictly keto: No modifications needed.

Berry Power Smoothie

1 cup unsweetened almond or coconut milk, or more as needed

¼ cup frozen or fresh blueberries, raspberries, or strawberries

¼ cup clementine segments or fresh plums

2 tablespoons unsweetened cashew butter

1 tablespoon ground flaxseed or chia seeds

1 tablespoon avocado oil

1 scoop Keto Zone vanilla hydrolyzed collagen powder

1–2 teaspoons stevia (debittered) or monk fruit sweetener (optional)

Splash of vanilla extract (optional)

Dash of ground cinnamon (optional)

Place all ingredients in a blender and process until smooth and creamy, adding more almond milk as needed to achieve your desired consistency. (1 serving)

Mediterranean-keto:

Calories: 487; net carbs: 19 grams

Strictly keto: Use macadamia nut butter or almond butter in place of cashew butter. Do not add clementine segments or plums.

Calories: 452; net carbs: 7 grams

Green Deviled Eggs

> 4 large hard-boiled eggs
> 1 avocado, chopped
> 2 tablespoons lemon juice
> 1–2 tablespoons extra-virgin olive oil
> 1 clove garlic, minced
> 1 red chili pepper, seeded and minced
> Salt and pepper to taste
> 4 slices cooked turkey bacon or pork bacon (nitrate/nitrite free), crumbled
> 1 tablespoon minced fresh chives

Halve eggs lengthwise. Gently scoop out the yolks and mash them with the avocado. Mix in the lemon juice, olive oil, garlic, chili pepper, salt, and pepper. Spoon the mixture back into the egg white halves. Top with bacon and chives, and serve chilled. Makes 8 deviled eggs. Suggested serving: 4 deviled eggs for women, 6 deviled eggs for men.

Mediterranean-keto:

> **Each deviled egg**—calories: 99; net carbs: 1 gram

Strictly keto: No modifications needed.

Hearty Vegetable Frittata

> 2 large eggs (3 for men)
> 1 tablespoon fresh chopped or ½ teaspoon dried herbs, such as rosemary, thyme, oregano, basil
> Salt and pepper to taste
> 1 tablespoon avocado oil
> ½ cup chopped fresh spinach, arugula, kale, or other leafy greens
> 2 ounces artichoke hearts, quartered, rinsed, drained, and dried
> 4 cherry tomatoes, cut in half
> 1 tablespoon diced black or Kalamata olives
> ¼ cup crumbled soft goat or feta cheese
> 1 tablespoon extra-virgin olive oil (2 tablespoons for men)

Preheat the oven to broil on low. Whisk eggs, herbs, salt, and pepper in a small bowl. Heat avocado oil over medium heat in a small oven-safe skillet or omelet pan. Add the spinach, artichoke hearts, and cherry tomatoes, and sauté 1–2 minutes. Add the egg mixture and let it cook undisturbed over medium heat for 3 to 4 minutes, until bottom begins to set. Sprinkle the olives and cheese on the egg mixture. Transfer the skillet to the oven to broil for 4–5 minutes, or until the frittata is firm in the center and golden on top. Remove from the oven. With a spatula, loosen the frittata from the sides of the pan. Gently flip it onto a plate or platter. Drizzle with the olive oil. (1 serving)

Mediterranean-keto:

2 eggs with 1 tablespoon olive oil—calories: 511; net carbs: 5 grams

3 eggs with 2 tablespoons olive oil—calories: 702; net carbs: 5 grams

Strictly keto: No modifications needed.

Keto Zone Coffee

6–8 ounces brewed hot coffee
1–2 tablespoons MCT oil powder
¼–½ teaspoon stevia (debittered)
1–2 tablespoons macadamia nut oil (for buttery, nutty flavor)
½–1 teaspoon dark unsweetened cocoa powder (optional)
1 scoop Keto Zone chocolate hydrolyzed collagen (optional)

Place all the ingredients in a blender and process until smooth and foamy. Or briskly stir the oil, stevia, and cocoa powder into hot coffee. (1 serving)

Mediterranean-keto:

Calories: 271; net carbs: 0 grams

Strictly keto: No modifications needed.

LUNCHES

Avocado and Tomato Salad

2 tablespoons extra-virgin olive oil
1 teaspoon lemon juice (or to taste)
1 clove garlic, minced
¼ cup basil, torn
1 avocado, chopped
½ cup chopped tomato

1 tablespoon walnuts or pecans, chopped
Salt and pepper to taste
1 ½ cups fresh spinach or greens

Whisk oil, lemon, and garlic. In a separate bowl, combine basil, avocado, tomato, and walnuts. Toss with oil mixture. Season with salt and pepper. If you'd like to add protein, toss in chunks of cooked fish, shrimp, chicken, or steak. Serve over greens. (1 serving)

Mediterranean-keto:

Calories: 545; net carbs: 7 grams

Strictly keto: No modifications needed, but women will need to add minimal (1–2 ounces) or no protein to keep from exceeding the recommended calories per meal.

Garlicky Shrimp and Asian Cucumbers

SHRIMP:

2 tablespoons sesame oil
1 tablespoon reduced-sodium, gluten-free soy or tamari
   sauce or liquid aminos (such as Bragg's)
4 cloves garlic, minced
1 teaspoon arrowroot powder
1 tablespoon fish sauce (optional)
2 tablespoons avocado oil
1 pound wild raw shrimp, peeled and deveined, tails on
2 green onions, minced

ASIAN CUCUMBER SALAD:

2 cups sliced cucumbers
¼ cup sliced sweet onions
½ cup cooked green peas
2 tablespoons sesame oil
1 tablespoon apple cider vinegar
2 teaspoons sesame seeds
1 garlic clove, minced
Salt and pepper to taste

Whisk sesame oil, soy sauce, garlic, arrowroot, and fish sauce until smooth. Set aside. Heat avocado oil over medium heat. Add shrimp and cook for 1–2 minutes per side. Pour sauce over shrimp. Simmer for 5 minutes. Top with green onions. Separately mix salad ingredients together. Serve shrimp with ¼ cup of cooked white basmati rice (51 calories; 11 grams net carbs) or quinoa (56 calories; 9 grams net carbs) and 1 cup salad. (2 servings)

Mediterranean-keto:

> **Shrimp dish without sides** (6 ounces)—calories: 474; net carbs: 4 grams

> **Salad** (1 cup)—calories: 194; net carbs: 9 grams

Strictly keto: Omit peas from side salad. Serve shrimp without rice or quinoa. To stay within optimal calorie range, women have 4 ounces of shrimp and men have 6–8 ounces of shrimp.

> **Shrimp dish** (4 ounces)—calories: 316; net carbs: 2 grams

> **Salad** (1 cup)—calories: 163; net carbs: 3 grams

Chili-Spiced Salmon Over Wilted Spinach

SALMON:

> 3 to 6 ounces wild salmon
> 1 tablespoon extra-virgin olive oil
> ¼ teaspoon garlic powder or to taste
> ¼ teaspoon chili powder or to taste
> Salt and pepper to taste
> Juice of ½ lemon

SPINACH:

> 1 tablespoon grass-fed ghee
> 1 10-ounce bag baby spinach
> 1 garlic clove, minced
> 2 tablespoons extra-virgin olive oil
> Juice of ½ lemon
> Salt and pepper to taste
> ¼ cup gluten-free pasta (optional)

Brush salmon with olive oil. Sprinkle with garlic powder, chili powder, salt, and pepper. Grill over medium heat until fish flakes easily with fork. Remove from heat, and drizzle with lemon juice and olive oil.

Heat ghee in a large skillet over low heat. Add the spinach and cook until just wilted. Add the garlic, salt, and pepper, and cook 1 minute. Remove from heat. Drizzle with olive oil and lemon.

Break up salmon into bite-size pieces. Toss with spinach and serve with ¼ cup of gluten-free garbanzo/chickpea pasta if desired. Sprinkle with extra lemon juice, olive oil, salt, and pepper as needed. (1 serving)

Mediterranean-keto:

> Calories (with 6 ounces salmon): 781; net carbs: 6 grams (Add 190 calories and 24 grams net carbs if you serve with gluten-free chickpea pasta, such as the Banza brand.)

Strictly keto: Omit the gluten-free pasta; serve salmon over the spinach. I recommend women have 3 ounces of salmon and drizzle only 1 tablespoon of olive oil over spinach. This will result in 540 calories and 6 grams of net carbs.

Seeded Bread Sandwiches

BREAD:

3 tablespoons ground chia seeds
3 tablespoons ground psyllium seeds
¾ cup raw sunflower seeds
¾ cup ground flaxseeds
1 cup ground hemp seeds
¾ cup ground pumpkin seeds
1 teaspoon salt
½ teaspoon stevia (1 packet)
1½ cups water
1½ tablespoons avocado oil
1½ tablespoons grass-fed ghee, melted

SANDWICH FILLINGS:

Nitrate-/nitrite-free ham or turkey
Avocado wedges
Sliced tomato
Sliced cucumber
Hummus
Feta cheese
Avocado oil mayonnaise
Yellow or stone-ground mustard

Combine seeds, salt, and stevia in a large bowl. In a separate bowl, whisk together the water, oil, and ghee. Pour the liquid mixture into the seed mixture. Mix well. Let stand for 2 to 3 hours. Preheat the oven to 350 degrees. Line a loaf pan with parchment paper. Pour batter into the pan, and bake 70–80 minutes. Cool completely, then slice for sandwiches. Makes 10 slices. (10 servings)

Build sandwiches with fillings of choice, staying mindful of your macros. Serve sandwich with a side of guacamole and a few (four or five) cassava chips.

Mediterranean-keto:

Calories per slice: 298; net carbs: 0.5 grams

Nitrate/nitrite-free ham or turkey (60–70 calories; 2 grams net carbs per ounce); ¼ avocado (80 calories; 1 gram net carbs); sliced tomato (5 calories; 1 gram net carbs); sliced cucumber (5 calories; 1 gram net carbs); hummus (80 calories; 2 grams net carbs per 2 tablespoons); feta cheese (70 calories; 1 gram net carbs per ¼ cup); avocado oil mayonnaise (90–100 calories; 0 grams net carbs per tablespoon); yellow or stone-ground mustard (4 calories; 0 grams net carbs per tablespoon); guacamole (70 calories; 1 gram net carbs per 2 ounces)

Strictly keto: Serve guacamole with celery or jicama slices (49 calories; 5 grams net carbs per cup) instead of cassava chips. Make sure sandwich fillings don't exceed 200 calories. Women, use 1 slice of bread and make sandwich open-faced to keep calories between 450 and 600.

Keto Burgers and Sweet Potato Wedges

2 sweet potatoes, cut into wedges
1 tablespoon avocado or coconut oil
Salt and pepper
1 pound grass-fed ground beef
2 teaspoons garlic powder
1 teaspoon salt
½ teaspoon pepper
½ cup feta cheese
Romaine or butter lettuce
Tomato slices (optional)
Onion slices (optional)
Avocado slices (optional)
Mustard (optional)

Avocado oil mayo (optional)

Preheat oven to 400 degrees. Drizzle sweet potato wedges with avocado oil and season with salt and pepper. Bake for 15–20 minutes. While potatoes bake, add garlic powder, salt, and pepper to ground beef. Mix well then shape into 4 patties. Grill or broil the burger to desired doneness. When you flip the burgers, top each burger with feta cheese. Serve burgers between 2–4 lettuce leaves, topped with tomato, onion, mustard, mayo, and avocado. (4 servings)

Mediterranean-keto:

With sweet potato wedges but without burger toppings—calories: 413; net carbs: 14 grams

Strictly keto: Omit the sweet potato wedges. Instead, serve with a side salad made with 1 cup lettuce, ½ avocado, 1 tablespoon olive oil, 1 teaspoon vinegar, and lemon juice to taste (241 calories; 2 grams net carbs) or a side salad made with lettuce, tomato, cucumbers, 1 tablespoon olive oil, and 1 teaspoon vinegar (145 calories; 4 grams net carbs). Men may add another 2 tablespoons olive oil to add 240 calories.

Burger without toppings or side salad—calories: 325; net carbs: 2 grams

Cilantro Chicken Soup

1 (3–4 pound) free-range chicken, skin removed; 14 ounces frozen grilled chicken fajita strips; or whole rotisserie chicken
Organic chicken broth (enough to cover chicken, 1–2 quarts)
Himalayan salt to taste
1 cup onions, chopped
1 cup mushrooms, chopped
1 cup broccoli, chopped
¼–½ cup peppers (optional)
¼–½ cup fresh cilantro, chopped
6–8 tablespoons extra-virgin olive oil or avocado oil
½–1 cup white basmati rice, cooked

Place the chicken, enough broth to cover chicken, and salt in a slow cooker. Cook on low for 3–4 hours. (To save cooking time, you can also cook the chicken in a stockpot on the stove. Bring to a boil, reduce to a simmer, and cook for 1 hour 15 minutes. Then reduce heat to low.) Remove chicken from the cooker or pot and let sit until cool enough to handle. Pull chicken from bones in bite-size pieces. Return chicken meat to cooker or pot. Add vegetables, cilantro, oil, and rice 15 to 30 minutes before serving so they don't get too soft. Ladle soup into bowls in 1½-cup portions. (4 servings)

For a faster soup, use a rotisserie chicken and remove skin and pull meat off bones in bite-size pieces, or use frozen grilled chicken fajita strips. Put meat in pot on stovetop with enough broth to cover the chicken. Bring to a boil, then simmer for 20 to 30 minutes. Add veggies, cilantro, olive oil, and rice, and simmer until veggies are softened. If desired, serve with a side salad made with 1 cup lettuce, 4 slices tomato, 1 tablespoon olive oil, 1 teaspoon apple cider vinegar, salt, pepper, and lemon juice to taste (195 calories; 3 grams net carbs).

Mediterranean-keto:

> **1 ½ cups**—calories: 549; net carbs: 18 grams

Strictly keto: Omit rice. Men add 1–2 tablespoons olive oil to add another 120–240 calories.

> **1 ½ cups**—calories: 489; net carbs: 5 grams

Chicken or Tongol Tuna Salad on Greens

SALAD:

> 3–4 tablespoons avocado oil mayo
> ¼ cup chopped celery
> ¼ cup chopped onions
> 3–6 ounces cooked chopped chicken or (low-mercury) tongol tuna[1]
> Celery seed, celery salt, garlic or garlic salt (optional)
> Salt and pepper to taste
> Any mix of butter lettuce, arugula, field greens, or spinach
> ¼ cup sliced cucumbers
> ¼ cup sliced tomatoes
> ½ cup white or garbanzo beans
> 1 tablespoon sunflower seeds
> ¼ cup feta or soft goat cheese, crumbled

---

1 Tongol tuna, which can be found at health-food stores, is very low in mercury.

OIL AND VINEGAR DRESSING:

¼ cup apple cider vinegar
¾ cup extra-virgin olive oil or avocado oil
Onion juice to taste
Minced garlic or garlic powder to taste
Dried oregano to taste
Salt and pepper to taste

Combine mayo, celery, onion, chicken/tuna, salt, pepper, and spices. Mix well. Fill salad bowl with greens. Top with vegetables, beans, sunflower seeds, then chicken/tuna salad. Whisk dressing ingredients together, and drizzle a few tablespoons over salad. Sprinkle with feta or goat cheese. You also may substitute butter lettuce for greens and put chicken/tuna salad between 2 butter lettuce leaves and eat as a sandwich. (1 serving)

Mediterranean-keto:

Salad with 6 ounces meat—calories: 644; net carbs: 20 grams

Dressing per 2 tablespoons—calories: 180; net carbs: 0 grams

Strictly keto: Omit beans from salad recipe. I recommend 3 ounces chicken or tuna for women and 6 ounces for men.

Salad with 3 ounces meat—calories: 397; net carbs: 7 grams

Salad with 6 ounces meat—calories: 540; net carbs: 7 grams

Keto-Friendly Chili

2 pounds grass-fed ground beef
2 tablespoons avocado oil
1 medium yellow onion, chopped
3 to 4 cloves garlic, minced
1 tablespoon tomato paste
2 tablespoons chili powder
2 teaspoons ground cumin
1 can (14-ounce) diced tomatoes
⅓ cup water
1 can (14-ounce) black, pinto, or kidney beans
1 green bell pepper, diced (optional)
Sliced green onions (optional)
Sliced jalapeños (optional)
Cilantro (optional)

In a large pot, brown the ground beef. Drain the meat, reserving half of the drippings. Set aside meat. Add oil to drippings and heat pan. If desired, add bell pepper, onion, and garlic, and cook until lightly browned. Stir in tomato paste, chili powder, and cumin. Cook for 1 minute. Add water, tomatoes, and ground beef. Stir to combine. Bring to boil, then lower heat to a gentle simmer and cook for 1–2 hours. (Alternatively: After browning meat, transfer to a slow cooker and add remaining ingredients, except beans and toppings. Cook 4–6 hours.) Add beans and warm through. Top with green onions, jalapeños, and cilantro as desired. (6 servings)

Mediterranean-keto:

1 cup—calories: 518; net carbs: 14 grams

Strictly keto: Omit beans. I recommend men add 1 or 2 tablespoons avocado oil or a green salad with tomatoes, onions, and Oil and Vinegar Dressing to increase calories.

1 cup—calories: 460; net carbs: 7 grams

Fajita Skewers

1 pound grass-fed steak, cut in cubes
1 large onion
1 green or red bell pepper
15–20 mushrooms
1 tablespoon chili powder
1½ teaspoons paprika
1 teaspoon ground cumin
½ teaspoon garlic powder
½ teaspoon salt
¼ cup avocado oil
Juice of 2 limes
6 skewers

Place the cubed steak in a large container and set aside. Cut onion and pepper into 1-inch chunks. Add onion, pepper, and mushrooms to container with steak.

In a small bowl, combine the spices, salt, oil and lime juice. Whisk well, and pour into the container with steak and veggies. Place lid on container, and gently shake to distribute marinade. Place in the refrigerator for 30 to 45 minutes, shaking container 2 times while marinating.

Preheat a grill to medium-high heat. Thread roughly 3 ounces of steak, along with peppers, onions, and mushrooms onto the skewers. Grill the ka-bobs for 7 to 10 minutes, turning halfway, until desired doneness on steak. Makes 6 skewers.

May eat with a salad made with 1 cup of romaine lettuce, ¼ cup each of tomatoes, onions, and cucumbers, and a simple dressing made with 2 table-spoons of extra-virgin olive oil and 2 teaspoons of vinegar. (277 calories; 6 grams net carbs)

Mediterranean-keto:

> **1 skewer**—calories: 201; net carbs: 5 grams

Strictly keto: Omit one vegetable to reduce carbs. Suggested serving: 2 skewers for women and 3 for men.

> **1 skewer**—calories: 191; net carbs: 3 grams

Keto Cobb Salad

> 3 cups mixed greens
> 3–6 ounces cooked pasture-raised chicken or turkey
> 1 slice cooked bacon or turkey bacon, diced
> 1 large egg, hard-boiled and sliced
> 4 grape tomatoes, halved
> ½ avocado, sliced or cubed
> ¼ cup sliced mushrooms
> 2 tablespoons low-carb ranch dressing (made with avocado
>   or extra-virgin olive oil such as Primal Kitchen's ranch
>   dressing)
> ¼ cup soft goat or feta cheese crumbles (optional)

Place greens in a large bowl. Add chicken or turkey, bacon, egg, tomatoes, avocado, and mushrooms. Top with dressing and cheese. (1 serving)

Mediterranean-keto:

> **With cheese and 6 ounces chicken or turkey**—calories: 747; net carbs: 7 grams

Strictly keto: No modifications needed, but I recommend women use 3 ounces meat and ½ ounce cheese to remain within their calorie limits.

> **With 2 tablespoons cheese and 3 ounces chicken or turkey**—calories: 560; net carbs: 7 grams

DINNERS

Asian Stir Fry

    1½ tablespoons avocado oil

    1½ tablespoons sesame seed oil

    3–6 ounces chicken cut into bite-size pieces

    2 cups veggies (broccoli, cabbage, bok choy, green onion, peppers, mushrooms)

    1 garlic clove, minced

    ½ tablespoon fresh ginger, minced

    1 teaspoon organic soy sauce (gluten-free, non-GMO) or tamari sauce

    Chili garlic sauce to taste

    Sesame seeds

    1 green onion, minced

    ¼ cup cooked basmati rice

Heat the avocado and sesame seed oils in a large skillet over medium heat. Add the chicken, turning after 3–4 minutes. Cook until almost done. Add vegetables, garlic, and ginger and cook until tender-crisp, stirring occasionally. Remove from heat. Drizzle with avocado oil and gluten-free soy sauce. Dot with chili garlic sauce for spiciness. Sprinkle with sesame seeds and green onion. Serve over rice. (1 serving)

Mediterranean-keto:

    With 6 ounces chicken—calories: 860; net carbs: 33 grams

Strictly keto: Omit rice. Women use 3 ounces of chicken and 1 tablespoon each of the sesame seed and avocado oils to stay within their calorie limits. Men use 6 ounces of chicken.

    With 3 ounces chicken, 1 tablespoon sesame seed oil, and 1 tablespoon avocado oil—calories: 515; net carbs: 7 grams

    With 6 ounces chicken—calories: 741; net carbs: 7 grams

Shrimp Scampi

    1 tablespoon grass-fed ghee

    4 tablespoons avocado oil, divided

    4–8 ounces raw wild shrimp, peeled

    1 clove garlic, minced

Juice of ½ lemon
2 tablespoons dry white wine
Salt and pepper to taste
1–2 cups asparagus or broccoli

Heat the ghee and 3 tablespoons avocado oil in a skillet over medium heat. When melted, add the shrimp. Turn shrimp once, and cook until pink throughout, about 3 minutes. Add the garlic, lemon, wine, salt, and pepper. Cook 1 minute. Remove from pan. Heat remaining oil. Sauté asparagus or broccoli for 3–4 minutes. Season with salt and pepper. (1 serving)

Mediterranean-keto:

With 8 ounces shrimp—calories: 875; net carbs: 7 grams

Strictly keto: Omit wine from sauce and use no more than 1½ cups of veggies. Women use 4 ounces of shrimp and cook it in 1 tablespoon of ghee and 2 tablespoons of avocado oil. Men use 8 ounces of shrimp and cook it in 1 tablespoon of ghee and 3 tablespoons of avocado oil.

With modifications for women—calories: 497; net carbs: 6 grams

With modifications for men—calories: 717; net carbs: 6 grams

Mediterranean-Keto Pizza

CRUST:

¼ cup coconut flour, sifted
¼ teaspoon salt
½ teaspoon herbs and spices (any mixture of basil, thyme, garlic powder, oregano, red pepper flakes, etc.)
2 tablespoons ground psyllium husks
1 tablespoon avocado or extra-virgin olive oil
1 cup warm water (not boiling)

SAUCE:

½ cup low-sugar tomato sauce
1 teaspoon herbs and spices (basil, thyme, garlic powder, oregano, red pepper flakes)
1 tablespoon extra-virgin olive oil

TOPPINGS:

Olives
Nitrate/nitrite-free sliced ham or cooked chicken strips

Artichoke hearts
Roasted red peppers
Mushrooms
Onions
½ cup goat cheese or feta crumbles or part-skim mozzarella
   cheese
¼ cup pine nuts, toasted
Fresh herbs (basil, oregano, thyme)

Preheat the oven to 400°F. Line a large baking sheet with parchment paper. In a large mixing bowl, combine coconut flour, salt, herbs/spices, psyllium husks, oil, and water. Mix well then knead the dough for 2 to 3 minutes. The batter may seem a little wet, but that's OK. Set dough aside for 15 minutes. Meanwhile, combine tomato sauce, herbs/spices, and 1 tablespoon olive oil. Sprinkle coconut or almond flour on counter or rolling sheet. Roll the dough out to ½-inch thickness. Place on baking sheet. Top crust with tomato sauce and toppings of choice. Bake for 12 to 15 minutes, or until the edges of the crust are slightly brown. Garnish with toasted pine nuts and fresh herbs. (2 servings)

Mediterranean-keto:

½ pizza—calories: 599; net carbs: 14 grams

Strictly keto: Omit pine nuts and use smaller amounts of the veggies. If desired, add a green side salad made with 1 cup lettuce, ½ avocado, 1 tablespoon olive oil, 1 teaspoon vinegar, and lemon juice to taste (241 calories; 2 grams net carbs) or with spinach, goat or feta cheese, 1 tablespoon olive oil, and 1 teaspoon vinegar (165 calories; 1 gram net carbs). Men add 1 more ounce feta or goat cheese (75–80 calories; 1–2 grams net carbs per ounce) and/or 1–2 tablespoons olive oil (120–240 calories) if needed to increase calories.

½ pizza—calories: 375; net carbs: 7 grams

Tip: This pizza has a few extra carbs, so lower the carbs on your other meals to account for them. If you don't want to make your own pizza crust, buy a low-carb cauliflower-crust pizza. There are several brands that are very low in net carbs. For instance, the Cali'flour brand's traditional flavor has 90 calories and 1 gram of net carbs per serving. (If you have a hard time digesting cauliflower, take an alpha-galactosidase enzyme product such as Beano before you eat to prevent stomach upset.) I like to put olive oil on the crust, then pizza sauce, then goat or part-skim mozzarella cheese. Then I add toppings: lots of mushrooms and onions, a small amount of ham, then a little minced garlic on top. That makes a delicious pizza!

Chinese Chicken Strips

⅓ cup quinoa
1 cup coconut milk
1 cup water
Cilantro to taste
Green onions, sliced
4 tablespoons organic gluten-free soy sauce (non-GMO)
4 tablespoons rice vinegar
½ teaspoon sesame oil
1 teaspoon red pepper flakes
4 tablespoons chicken broth
½ teaspoon ground ginger
½ teaspoon onion powder
6 boneless skinless chicken breasts, cut into strips
2 eggs
1 cup almond flour
3 tablespoons avocado oil

Cook quinoa according to package instructions, using coconut milk for half of the liquid and water for the remaining half. When quinoa is ready, stir in cilantro and green onions. Serve in ¼-cup portions.

To prepare the meat, whisk soy, vinegar, ½ teaspoon of sesame oil, red pepper flakes, chicken broth, ginger, and onion powder in a bowl. Add chicken and marinate for 30 minutes up to 2 hours. In a separate bowl, whisk the eggs. Pour the almond flour onto a shallow plate. Drain marinade. Dip chicken pieces into the almond flour, coating all sides, and then dip it into the egg mixture. Heat avocado oil in large pan over medium heat. Cook chicken for 7–8 minutes, turning strips halfway, until brown and cooked through. Garnish with green onions. Serve with quinoa and a side of sautéed vegetables such as cabbage or broccoli. (4–6 servings)

Mediterranean-keto:

> **With 6 ounces chicken**—calories: 761; net carbs: 15 grams

Strictly keto: Omit quinoa. Increase amount of sautéed vegetables on the side to 1 cup. Suggested serving: 4 ounces chicken for women and 6 ounces for men.

> **With 4 ounces chicken**—calories: 491; net carbs: 6 grams

> **With 6 ounces chicken**—calories: 652; net carbs: 6 grams

Curried Shrimp and Broccoli

> 1 tablespoon avocado oil
> 1 tablespoon extra-virgin coconut oil
> 1 pound raw wild shrimp, peeled
> 1 tablespoon yellow curry powder
> ¼ teaspoon cinnamon
> Salt and pepper to taste
> 2 oranges, seeded and quartered
> ½ cup snap peas, cut in half
> Fresh cilantro
> 1 tablespoon extra-virgin olive oil
> 2 cups broccoli, chopped
> Salt and pepper to taste
> Lemon wedges

Heat avocado and coconut oils in a skillet over medium heat. Add shrimp and cook for about 2 minutes per side. Add curry powder, cinnamon, salt, pepper, orange pieces, and peas, stirring well. Cook until shrimp are pink and start to curl and oranges are browned. Garnish with fresh cilantro before serving.

In a separate pan, heat olive oil and cook broccoli until tender, stirring occasionally. Season with salt, pepper, and lemon juice. (2 servings)

Mediterranean-keto:

> **With 6 ounces curried shrimp**—calories: 498; net carbs: 20 grams

Strictly keto: Omit snap peas and oranges. Add 1 cup cabbage sautéed in 1 tablespoon olive oil (132 calories; 1.6 grams net carbs). Men can cook 2 cups veggies in 2 tablespoons olive oil to add 264 calories and 3.2 grams net carbs.

> **With 6 ounces curried shrimp**—calories: 433; net carbs: 5 grams

Stuffed Pork Chops

1 slice cooked bacon (nitrate/nitrite free), diced
½ cup chopped white mushrooms
2 ounces goat cheese, crumbled
1 teaspoon chopped fresh rosemary
1 large clove garlic, minced
2 (12-ounce) bone-in pork chops (about 1 inch thick)
½ teaspoon salt
¼ teaspoon pepper
¼ teaspoon garlic powder
1 tablespoon avocado oil

Preheat the oven to 350 degrees. In a small bowl mix bacon, mushrooms, goat cheese, rosemary, and garlic. Cut a large slit in the side of each pork chop. Do not cut all the way through. Stuff the pork chops with the mushroom filling, then press closed and secure with toothpicks or twine. Season the chops with salt, pepper, and garlic powder.

Heat the avocado oil in an oven-safe pan over medium-high heat. Sear each side of the pork chops, about 2 to 3 minutes per side. Transfer the pan to the oven and bake for 25 to 30 minutes. Internal meat temperature should reach 145 degrees. Allow the pork chops to rest for 3 to 5 minutes before serving. Serve with ½ cup roasted yams and a side salad made with lettuce, tomato, cucumbers, 1 tablespoon olive oil, and 1 teaspoon vinegar. (2 servings)

Mediterranean-keto:

Including yams and salad—calories: 788; net carbs: 20 grams

Strictly Keto: Suggested serving: 8 ounces of pork for women and 12 ounces for men. Omit yams. Serve with a salad made with 2 cups lettuce, ½ cup tomatoes, ½ cup cucumbers, 2 tablespoons olive oil, and 2 teaspoons vinegar (279 calories; 5 grams net carbs) and/or 1 cup green beans sautéed in 2 tablespoons olive oil (271 calories; 4 grams net carbs). Men may add 1–2 tablespoons olive oil if needed to increase calories.

6 ounces pork—calories: 281; net carbs: 1 gram

8 ounces pork—calories: 375; net carbs: 1 gram

Garlic Steak and Cauliflower Rice

2 grass-fed rib eye steaks, 3 ounces each
1 tablespoon grass-fed ghee, divided
1 tablespoon avocado oil, divided
2 cloves garlic, minced
1 medium head cauliflower
2 tablespoons extra-virgin olive oil
1 clove garlic, minced
Salt and pepper

Grill or pan sear rib eyes over medium heat until desired doneness. In a small pan, melt the ghee; then add the garlic and avocado oil. Cook for 1 minute. Drizzle ghee and avocado oil over top of steaks.

Core the cauliflower and chop coarsely. Pulse cauliflower in food processor until it looks like large pieces of rice. In a large skillet over medium heat, heat the olive oil. Add the garlic and sauté for 1 minute. Add the riced cauliflower and cook for about 10 minutes or until the cauliflower rice is tender. Season with salt and pepper. (2 servings)

Mediterranean-keto:

> **6 ounces steak and 2 cups cauliflower rice**—calories: 501; net carbs: 10 grams

Strictly keto: Limit cauliflower rice to 1 cup. Add green salad made with 1 cup lettuce, ½ avocado, 1 tablespoon olive oil, 1 teaspoon vinegar, and lemon juice to taste. Suggested serving: 4 ounces steak for women and 6 ounces for men.

> **4 ounces steak with cauliflower rice and salad**—calories: 542; net carbs: 7 grams

> **6 ounces steak with cauliflower rice and salad**—calories: 644; net carbs: 7 grams

Macadamia Nut-Crusted Wild Tilapia

2 (4-ounce) wild tilapia fillets
½ cup unsalted macadamia nuts
1 tablespoon chopped fresh parsley
1 tablespoon fresh lemon juice
2 tablespoons avocado oil
¼ teaspoon garlic powder

Salt and pepper to taste
2 tablespoons olive oil
Lemon wedges, for serving

Preheat the oven to 400 degrees. Line a rimmed baking sheet with parchment paper. Place the nuts, parsley, and lemon juice in a food processor and pulse until the mixture is combined and looks like crumbs. Spread mixture onto a plate.

Brush each fillet with avocado oil. Then press both sides of the fish into the nut mixture. Sprinkle with garlic, salt, and pepper. Bake for 10 to 15 minutes, until the top is crisp and slightly golden brown. Squeeze lemon over the top before serving. Serve with a side salad, cauliflower rice, or sautéed bok choy. (2 servings)

Serve with cauliflower rice (100 calories; 5 grams net carbs), sautéed bok choy (90 calories; 2 grams net carbs), a side salad made with 1 cup lettuce, ½ avocado, 1 tablespoon olive oil, 1 teaspoon vinegar, and lemon juice to taste (241 calories; 2 grams net carbs) or with lettuce, tomato, cucumbers, 1 tablespoon olive oil, and 1 teaspoon vinegar (145 calories; 4 grams net carbs).

Mediterranean-keto:

4-ounce fillet only—calories: 480; net carbs: 3 grams

Strictly keto: No modifications needed.

Zoodles

2 to 3 medium zucchinis
1 tablespoon grass-fed ghee
3 tablespoons extra-virgin olive oil
1 small clove garlic, pressed
Italian herbs (optional)
Salt and pepper

Rinse the zucchini and cut off both ends. Push the zucchini through a spiral slicer (spiralizer). Heat ghee and oil in a large skillet over medium heat. Add garlic and cook for 1 minute. Add the zucchini noodles and Italian herbs. Toss to coat in the garlic butter. Cook for 1 to 5 minutes to desired doneness. Season with salt and pepper. Serve with protein of choice or as a side to any dish. (2 servings)

Mediterranean-keto:

1 cup—calories: 237; net carbs: 1 gram

Strictly keto: No modifications needed.

Red Curry Chicken

2 tablespoons avocado oil
1 pound boneless, skinless chicken thighs
1 green bell pepper, sliced
1 red bell pepper, sliced
1 cup snap peas, sliced in half
1 can (14-ounce) coconut milk
1 tablespoon fish sauce (optional)
2 tablespoons red curry paste
8–10 fresh basil leaves, sliced
Salt and pepper to taste
Red pepper flakes (optional)

Heat the oil in a large skillet over medium heat. Add the chicken. Cook for 3–4 minutes per side. Remove chicken and set aside. Add bell peppers and snap peas to pan. Cook until the peppers are tender. Remove from the pan and set aside. In the same skillet, combine the coconut milk, fish sauce, and curry paste. Stir well to combine and simmer for 4 to 5 minutes. Chop the chicken into bite-sized pieces. Add chicken, peppers, peas, and basil leaves to pan. Stir and simmer for 3 to 4 minutes. Season with salt, pepper, and chili flakes. Serve over cauliflower rice if desired (100 calories; 5 grams net carbs). (3 servings)

Mediterranean-keto:

With 6 ounces chicken—calories: 698; net carbs: 12 grams

Strictly keto: Omit snap peas. Add broccoli or mushrooms instead. Suggested serving: 4 ounces chicken for women and 6 ounces chicken for men.

With 4 ounces chicken—calories: 348; net carbs: 6 grams

With 6 ounces chicken—calories: 458; net carbs: 7 grams

SNACKS AND DESSERTS

Cauliflower Hummus

> 1 tablespoon grass-fed ghee
> 1 medium cauliflower, chopped finely
> 3–4 garlic cloves
> 2 tablespoons lemon or lime juice
> 6 tablespoons tahini
> 3 tablespoons extra-virgin olive oil or avocado oil, plus
>   more if needed
> ¼ teaspoon cumin
> Salt and pepper to taste

Heat ghee in a sauté pan over medium heat. Add the cauliflower and cook until tender. Add garlic and cook for 1–2 minutes, stirring constantly. Remove from heat and cool. Place in a food processor or blender, add remaining ingredients, and pulse until smooth, regularly scraping down the sides. If too thick, add an extra tablespoon of olive oil or water until you reach preferred consistency. Makes roughly 2 cups. (6 servings)

Mediterranean-keto:

⅓-cup serving—calories: 194; net carbs: 6 grams

Strictly keto: No modifications needed.

Zingy Avocado Dip

> 2 medium avocados
> 1½ teaspoons lemon juice
> ¼ teaspoon red pepper flakes
> Garlic powder, onion powder, or cumin (optional)
> Fresh chopped cilantro (optional)
> Salt and pepper to taste

In a food processor, blend all ingredients until smooth. Serve with sliced peppers, celery, or jicama. This dip will keep in the fridge for up to 3 days. (4 servings)

Mediterranean-keto:

½-cup serving—calories: 117; net carbs: 2 grams

Strictly keto: No modifications needed.

Nutty Granola Bars

½ cup chopped almonds
1 tablespoon chia seeds
6 tablespoons ground flaxseed meal
6 tablespoons mixed seeds (sunflower, pumpkin, sesame, etc.)
½ teaspoon debittered stevia (or to taste)
¼ cup shredded coconut
Pinch salt
¼ teaspoon cinnamon (optional)
½ cup almond butter (or any nut or seed butter)
¼ cup avocado oil

Line an 8-inch square pan with parchment paper. In a medium bowl, stir together the dry ingredients. In a small microwave-safe bowl, combine the almond butter and avocado oil. Heat 30 seconds to 1 minute. Whisk well. Pour into the dry mixture and stir well. Firmly press the batter into the pan. Refrigerate until firm. Cut into 12 bars. (12 servings)

Mediterranean-keto:

1 bar—calories: 181; net carbs: 2 grams

Strictly keto: Use macadamia nuts and macadamia nut butter in place of almonds and almond butter.

Smoked Salmon and Cucumber Bites

4 ounces goat cheese
2 tablespoons extra-virgin olive oil, plus extra for drizzling
1 tablespoon minced capers
1 tablespoon minced red onion
1 teaspoon dried dill
Red pepper flakes or chili powder (optional)
6 ounces smoked wild-caught Alaskan salmon (Biltmore is my favorite brand)
Cucumber slices (about a dozen)
Salt and pepper to taste

In a small bowl, combine the goat cheese, olive oil, capers, onion, dill, and red pepper flakes. Mix well. Cut smoked salmon into 1-inch pieces. Place one piece of salmon on each cucumber slice. Add dollop of goat cheese mixture on top. Drizzle with olive oil and sprinkle with salt and pepper. (4 servings)

Mediterranean-keto:

Calories: 287; net carbs: 1 gram

Strictly keto: No modifications needed.

Keto Crackers

> 1 cup almond flour
> 3 tablespoons small seeds of your liking (sesame seeds, flax-
> seeds, hemp seeds, fennel seeds)
> ¼ teaspoon baking soda
> Salt and pepper to taste
> 1 large egg, at room temperature
> 1 tablespoon extra-virgin olive oil

Preheat the oven to 350 degrees. Line a baking sheet with parchment paper. Combine dry ingredients in a large bowl. Stir well. In a small bowl, whisk the egg and olive oil. Pour into the dry ingredients. Mix well, then form a ball with the dough. Between pieces of parchment or plastic wrap, roll the dough to about ⅛ inch thick and shape into a rectangle. Cut the dough into 18 squares. Place onto baking sheet and bake for 10–15 minutes, until crispy and slightly golden. Store in an airtight container in the refrigerator for up to 4 days. Yields 18 crackers. One serving is 6 crackers.

Mediterranean-keto:

Calories: 236; net carbs: 4 grams

Strictly keto: No modifications needed.

Chocolate Peanut Butter Power Balls

> ¼ cup natural unsweetened almond butter or peanut butter
> ½ teaspoon stevia (debittered)
> 2 tablespoons blanched almond flour
> ¼ teaspoon vanilla extract
> 1 teaspoon flaxseeds
> ¼ cup sugar-free chocolate chips (such as Lilly's)
> 1½ teaspoons MCT oil

Line a plate with parchment paper. Mix all ingredients except chocolate chips and oil. Scoop peanut butter mixture into 10 balls and roll them between your hands. Place them on a parchment-lined plate and put in the freezer for 30 minutes. Melt chocolate chips in a small microwave-safe bowl and mix in the MCT oil. Remove the peanut butter balls from the freezer. Dip the balls one at a time into the melted chocolate. Place balls back on parchment-lined plate. Return to freezer for 10 minutes, until the chocolate is solid. Store in freezer for up to 6 months. (10 servings)

Mediterranean-keto:

> **1 ball**—calories: 66; net carbs: 3.2 grams

Strictly keto: Swap peanut butter for almond or mac nut butter.

> **1 ball**—calories: 66; net carbs: 2.7 grams

Frozen Lemon Cream

> ½ cup lemon juice
> 1–2 teaspoons stevia (debittered)
> 4 pastured organic eggs
> 4 tablespoons grass-fed ghee
> 4 tablespoons avocado oil
> 2 teaspoons unflavored grass-fed powdered gelatin

Combine all the ingredients in a saucepan. Heat over low heat until just before the mixture comes to a boil, but DO NOT boil. Cool slightly. Pour into ramekins or ice cube tray and freeze. Eat like ice cream in ½ cup servings (4 servings). If you have high cholesterol, use only 2 tablespoons of grass-fed ghee and 6 tablespoons of avocado oil.

Mediterranean-keto:

> Calories: 308; net carbs: 3 grams

Strictly keto: No modifications needed.

Chia Seed Pudding

> 1½ cups unsweetened vanilla almond, coconut, or oat milk
> 1 teaspoon stevia (debittered)
> ¼ cup chia seeds
> 1 teaspoon orange zest (optional)
> Blueberries, raspberries, or strawberries (optional)
> Sliced almonds (optional)

Whisk milk and sweetener well in a medium bowl. Add the chia seeds and mix well. Set aside for 10–15 minutes. Stir again to break up any chia seed clumps. Add orange zest if using. Cover and refrigerate overnight. Divide between two bowls or glasses. Serve topped with berries and nuts. Also great for breakfast! (2 servings)

Mediterranean-keto:

¾-cup serving (with toppings)—calories: 253; net carbs: 6 grams

Strictly keto: Use almond milk.

Keto Molten Lava Cake

2 ounces stevia-sweetened dark chocolate (at least 70 percent cacao)
2 ounces unsalted almond butter
2 pasture-raised eggs
1–2 teaspoons stevia (or to taste)
1 tablespoon super-fine almond flour

Heat oven to 350 degrees. Grease 2 ramekins with avocado oil.

Melt the chocolate and almond butter in a microwave-safe dish and stir well. In a separate bowl, beat eggs well with a mixer. Add eggs and sweetener to the chocolate mixture and mix well. Then add almond flour and stir until combined. Pour the batter into the ramekins. Bake for about 9 to 10 minutes. Let it sit 1 minute, then flip onto individual plates. Serve warm. (2 servings)

Mediterranean-keto:

1 cake—calories: 365; net carbs: 3 grams

Strictly keto: No modifications needed.

ADDITIONAL RESOURCES FOR LIVING IN THE HEALTH ZONE

N THIS APPENDIX, I list several tests I recommend patients request. This will help you know where you're starting and what areas you need to target to live in the Health Zone. Also included are several lists of supplements I recommend for the various phases of the journey.

TESTS

TESTS YOU CAN ASK YOUR DOCTOR TO REQUEST

Here are several of the levels I check and tests I request for many of my patients:

- levels of vitamin D_3 using 25-hydroxy (25 OH) vitamin D test

- vitamin B_{12} level

- inflammatory marker hs-CRP

- comprehensive metabolic panel

- complete blood count (CBC)

- lipid panel

- a cholesterol NMR (nuclear magnetic resonance) lipoprofile test, an oxidized LDL cholesterol test, and a lipoprotein(a) test if cholesterol levels remain elevated

- thyroid function by testing free T3, TSH, reverse T3, and TPO antibodies

- ferritin level (to check iron stores)

- hemoglobin A1c (which checks long-term blood sugar and insulin resistance)

- sex hormone levels for men (total and free testosterone and estradiol) and for women (FSH, estradiol, progesterone, and total and free testosterone)

Note: You don't need a blood test to start the healthy keto diet or the Mediterranean-keto lifestyle.

Note: When your weight loss stalls, this is often a good time to do thyroid tests, HbA1c tests to check for insulin resistance, and hs-CRP tests to check for chronic inflammation.

FOOD SENSITIVITY TEST

I recommend the Alcat Test to identify food sensitivities. To learn more, visit Cell Sciences Systems at cellsciencesystems.com/patients/alcat-test/ and cellsciencesystems.com/providers/alcat-test/.

The test measures non-IgE mediated reactions to food, chemicals, and other substances. "The Alcat Test is a lab based immune stimulation test in which a patient's WBC's are challenged with various substances including food, additives, colorings, chemicals, medicinal herbs, functional food, molds and pharmaceutical compounds....The Alcat Test objectively classifies a patient's response to each test substance as reactive, borderline or non-reactive. Based on these classifications, a customized elimination/rotation diet may be designed to effectively eliminate the specific triggers of chronic immune system activation."[1]

Hormone Lab Tests

Hormone health zone blood panel

- For men: TSH, free T3, total and free testosterone, SHBG, estradiol, rT3, TPO, and PSA

- For women: TSH, free T3, total and free testosterone, estradiol, rT3, TPO, FSH, and progesterone level

Divine health panel

- For men: all hormone tests for men, and CMP, CBC, HbA1c, hs-CRP, 25OHD$_3$ level, B$_{12}$ level, urinalysis, and lipid panel

- For women: all hormone tests for women and additional tests listed previously

- Adrenal testing: (1) DiagnosTechs Adrenal Panel at diagnostechs.com, (2) DHEA-S level, (3) salivary cortisol testing at 8:00 a.m., noon, 4:00 p.m., and 8:00 p.m.

Physician locator

- worldhealth.net
- biotemedical.com
- agemed.org
- brodabarnes.org

BLOOD TESTS FOR A HEALTHY BRAIN—AND THEIR TARGET VALUES

These are the most important initial blood tests for memory loss:

1. hs-CRP

2. hemoglobin A1c

3. homocysteine levels

4. ApoE gene testing

5. lipid panel

6. oxidized LDL cholesterol

7. vitamin B_{12} level

8. vitamin D_3 level ($25OHD_3$ level)

9. DHEA-S level

10. pregnenolone level

11. estradiol level

12. total and free testosterone level

13. free T3 level

14. TSH

15. MTHFR gene test

The following chart is a comprehensive list of all tests you may want to ask for. It also tells you where they're available, and most importantly, the target values you will want to compare with your individual results.

TARGET VALUES FOR TESTS ASSOCIATED WITH COGNITION

CATEGORY	TEST	LOCATION	TARGET VALUE
Inflammation	hs-CRP (high-sensitivity C-reactive protein)	Labcorp	<0.9 mg/dL
Insulin Resistance	Hemoglobin A1c percent	Labcorp	5.3 or less
	Fasting Glucose	Labcorp	70–90 mg/dL
	Fasting Insulin	Labcorp	<5.0 uIU/mL
Inflammation	Homocysteine Levels	Labcorp	≤ 7 mcmol/L
Alzheimer's	ApoE Alzheimer's Risk Testing	Labcorp	
	Omega-3 Index	Labcorp	a. ≥10 percent (ApoE4+) b. 8–10 percent (ApoE4-)
	Omega-6 to Omega-3 ratio	Labcorp	1 to 1 to 4 to 1 (Caution: <0.5 to 1 sometimes correlates with bleeding tendency.)
Cholesterol	LDL Particle Number	Labcorp	700–1200 nmol/L
	Small density LDL particle size	Labcorp	<121 mg/dL
	OxLDL (Oxidized LDL)	Labcorp	<60 ng/mL
	Total Cholesterol	Labcorp	150–200 mg/dL
	HDL	Labcorp	>50 mg/dL
	Triglycerides	Labcorp	<100 mg/dL
Minerals	RBC Magnesium	Labcorp	5.2–6.5 mg/dL
	Copper	Labcorp	90–110 mcg/dL
	Zinc	Labcorp	90–110 mcg/dL
Antioxidants	CoQ10	Labcorp	1.1–2.2 mcg/mL
	Glutathione	Labcorp	>250 mcg/mL
Vitamins	Vitamin B_{12}	Labcorp	500–1500 pg/mL
	Vitamin D_3	Labcorp	55–80 ng/mL
Genetics	MTHFR genetic test	Labcorp	If (+) with ≥ 1 mutation, need an active form of folic acid

CATEGORY	TEST	LOCATION	TARGET VALUE
Trophic factors (hormones)	Estradiol	Labcorp	20–50 pg/mL (Some women need higher levels.)
	FSH	Labcorp	23–50 IU/L
	Progesterone	Labcorp	1–20 ng/dL
	Pregnenolone	Labcorp	100–250 ng/dL
	Cortisol (AM)	Labcorp	10–18 mcg/dL
	DHEA-S level women	Labcorp	100–350 mcg/dL
	DHEA-S level men	Labcorp	150–500 mcg/dL
	Total Testosterone Men	Labcorp	500–1000 ng/dL
	Free Testosterone Men	Labcorp	15–26 pg/mL
	Total Testosterone Women	Labcorp	50–150 ng/dL (and even higher to 200 ng/dL for those female patients with osteoporosis or sarcopenia)
	Free T3	Labcorp	3.0–4.2 pg/mL
	Reverse T3	Labcorp	<20 ng/dL
	TSH	Labcorp	<2.0 mIU/L
	Anti-TPO	Labcorp	Negative
Toxins	Mercury	DoctorsData-Urine Metal Toxins. Optimal testing is done with urine, but serum blood testing is also available. Visit doctorsdata.com/Urine-Toxic-Metals and doctorsdata.com/Whole-Blood-Elements	a. Urine <0.8 mcg/g b. Blood <4.5 mcg/L
	Lead		a. Urine <1.1 mcg/g b. Blood <3.0 mcg/dL
	Arsenic		a. Urine <40 mcg/g b. Blood <9.0 mcg/L
	Cadmium		a. Urine <0.6 mcg/g b. Blood <1.0 mcg/L
	Benzene (optional) GPL-TOX Profile- urine	Great Plains Laboratory for optimal results. Also available from Labcorp and Quest Diagnostics.	Negative
	Toluene (optional)	Not available through Great Plains. It can be ordered through Labcorp or Quest Diagnostics.	Negative
	Glyphosate	Great Plains Laboratory	<1.0 mcg/g urinary creatinine
	C4a		<2830 ng/mL

CATEGORY	TEST	LOCATION	TARGET VALUE
Mold Toxins	Transforming Growth Factor Beta One (TGF-b1)		<2380 pg/mL
	MMP-9		85–332 ng/mL
	HLA Genotyping for Mold Susceptibility	www.survivingmold.com; Labcorp test code #167120 HLA genotyping (myhousemakesmesick.com/hlacalc)	Refer to Dr. Ritchie Shoemaker's protocol for specifics at www.survivingmold.com.
	MARCoNS Testing		Negative
	VCS Visual Contrast Sensitivity Screening	www.vcstest.com	
	MSH		35–81 pg/Ml
	ADH/osmolality		a. ADH 1.0–13.3 pg/mL b. Osmolality 280–300 mosmol
Pathogens	Antibodies to Lyme Disease: Bartonella	IGeneX laboratories	Negative
	Babesia	IGeneX laboratories	Negative
	Erlichia	IGeneX laboratories	Negative
	Antibodies to Herpes: a. HSV-1 IgM (chronic infection with reactivation of the virus may be a contributive factor to progressive brain damage characteristic of AD); IgG (dormant chronic infection is less likely)	IGeneX laboratories	Negative
	HSV-2 testing for this like above; however, HSV-2 rarely causes the progression to AD	IGeneX laboratories	Negative
	HHV-6	IGeneX laboratories	Negative

CATEGORY	TEST	LOCATION	TARGET VALUE
	VZV (Varicella Zoster Virus)	IGeneX laboratories	Negative
	EBV (Epstein-Barr Virus)	IGeneX laboratories	Negative
	CMV (Cytomegalovirus)	IGeneX laboratories	Negative
Sleep	Sleep study for nocturnal oxygen saturation		96–98 percent
Leaky gut and leaky brain	Leaky Gut Cyrex Array 2 (intestinal antigenic permeability screen)		
	Leaky Brain Cyrex Array 20 (blood-brain barrier permeability screen)		
Autoimmune testing	ANA titer and pattern		

SUPPLEMENTS

Divine Health supplements

Available at shop.drcolbert.com or by calling (407) 732-6952

- MCT oil powder—made of healthy fats that help support a healthy heart and brain. MCT oil also helps the liver produce ketone bodies, which assist the body into ketosis and set the body up to burn fat. Take about ½ teaspoon to 1 teaspoon of MCT oil powder in coffee or any hot liquid to avoid clumping, once or twice a day. Flavors include coconut cream, hazelnut, French vanilla, and chocolate.

- MCT oil capsules—have the MCT oil (1,000 milligrams) in capsule form to help you keep in ketosis. I call these MCT oil capsules "keto on the go." Take one or two capsules once or twice a day.

- High Potency Turmeric—with Bioperine for superior absorption. Turmeric is anti-inflammatory and binds to amyloid plaque in the brain and helps your body expel it. Bioperine increases its bioavailability by as much as 2,000 percent.

- Hormone Zone—contains DIM and synergistic nutrients that support healthy hormone (estradiol and free testosterone) levels in men and women

- Testosterone Zone—provides clinically studied ingredients, including synergistic nutrients and herbs that boost free testosterone levels naturally

- Thyroid Zone—a blend of nutrients and herbs designed specifically to support healthy thyroid function

- Fiber Zone—great-tasting psyllium husk powder with prebiotics (inulin), available flavors: berry or unflavored (contains soluble and insoluble fibers; I often recommend 1–2 tablespoons daily)

- Wild Alaskan Salmon omega-3 oil—each capsule contains 1000 milligrams of wild Alaskan salmon oil.

- Living Krill—two capsules contain 1000 milligrams of krill oil, with 200 milligrams of astaxanthin, and help protect the eyes and brain.

- Enhanced Multivitamin—contains the active forms of vitamins, including B vitamins, with chelated minerals for better absorption of the minerals

- Organic Green Supremefood—superfood drink with fourteen organic fermented veggies and grasses and no nightshades, with four different strains of probiotics and four digestive enzymes. It is fermented for better digestion and less gas.

- Organic Red Supremefood—contains nine organic fruits and is low sugar and includes raspberry, blueberry, cranberry, acai, and pomegranate

- Collagen powder—hydrolyzed collagen consists of chicken collagen, containing Type I and Type II collagen. As you age, your body slowly loses collagen throughout the body (hair, nails, joints, bones, heart, and skin). Your body's joints and skin repair at night, so it's best to take ½ to 1 scoop in any liquid thirty minutes before bed. Available in chocolate, vanilla, and unflavored.

- Divine Health Biotics—a powerful probiotic to help restore a leaky gut; contains *Bifidobacterium breve, Bifidobacterium lactis, Lactobacillus plantarum, Bacillus coagulans, Bacillus subtilis,* and the prebiotics fructooligosaccharides (FOS), and galactooligosaccharides (GOS). One veggie capsule contains sixteen billion CFUs (colony forming units) and 200 milligrams of prebiotics.

- Fat-Zyme—a digestive enzyme designed to break down fats and vegetables that is especially helpful for patients on a keto diet

- Brain Zone Basic—includes the active forms of the B vitamins—including methylated folate, methylcobalamin, and pyridoxal 5-phosphate in optimal dosages—curcumin, and TMG (trimethyl glycine) to lower homocysteine levels. (I especially recommend this for people with the MTHFR gene mutation and for patients with an elevated homocysteine level.)

- Brain Zone Advanced—a combination of nutritionals that boost BDNF (brain-derived neurotrophic factor) and NGF (neuro growth factor). These include 7,8 Dihydroxyflavone, lion's mane mushroom, lithium orotate, citicoline, and tyrosine. (I recommend this to patients experiencing mild, moderate, or severe memory loss. Start with one or two capsules at bedtime and gradually increase to one or two capsules two times a day.)

- Brain Zone Focus—powdered nutritionals that energize and fuel the brain. It contains D-ribose, alpha-GPC, taurine, N-acetyl tyrosine, green tea extract, and other nutrients to help one focus and energize the brain. Take this supplement in the morning and at noon but not at night because it energizes the brain and can cause insomnia if taken at night.

- Cellgevity—a glutathione-boosting supplement (To order, call 801-316-6380, code #231599.)

- Divine Health Carb Assist—a new supplement that supports healthy blood sugar levels by improving carbohydrate metabolism, insulin sensitivity, and the processing of dietary carbohydrates.

- Super Vitamin K_2—contains high-dose vitamin K_2, 200 milligrams per capsule, consisting of MK-7 for better bioavailability. Vitamin K_2 regulates calcium metabolism in the body, helping to build strong bones and preventing calcium buildup in the arteries, including cerebral arteries, thus supporting good blood flow to the brain.

- Divine Health Nano Glutathione—Glutathione is a powerful antioxidant often called "the master antioxidant" that combats inflammation, oxidative stress, infections, mental stress, toxins, and heavy metals in the body. Glutathione levels are being depleted by aging, toxin overload, poor diet, and stressed lifestyles. Nanotechnology offers rapid and more complete absorption from the GI tract.

- Q10 Vital—contains 100 milligrams of CoQ10, which is a crucial antioxidant for providing energy to all cells in the body. It is especially important for optimal cardiovascular health.

- Divine Health Refreshing Sleep Formula—contains natural supplements including GABA, magnesium glycinate, 5-HTP (5-hydroxytryptophan), L-theanine, melatonin, lemon balm extract, and ashwagandha, which helps one fall asleep and stay asleep.

Other recommended supplements

- Visbiome—for IBS, ulcerative colitis, and Crohn's disease; 112.5 billion CFU per capsule; available at www.visbiome.com (If a patient has severe leaky gut and dysbiosis, I commonly place him or her on two or more types of probiotics such as Divine Health Biotics and Visbiome.)

- MegaSporeBiotic—spore-based probiotic by Microbiome Labs that can form spores and is highly resistant to stomach acid; available at microbiomelabs.com/home/products/megasporebiotic

- Vitamin D_3—2,000 international units (IU)

- High-dose DHA—with a 2:1 ratio of DHA:EPA such as ProDHA 1000 from Nordic Naturals

- Magnesium threonate—144 milligrams per day or 350–400 milligrams of magnesium glycinate per day (It is best taken at night, as it helps you sleep.)

- Ketosis strips

To book an appointment with Dr. Colbert, call (407) 331-7007. Follow him on YouTube at Dr. Don Colbert MD, and tune into his podcast, *Divine Health With Dr. Don Colbert*, on the Charisma Podcast Network.

A PERSONAL NOTE FROM DON COLBERT, MD

GOD DESIRES TO heal you of disease. His Word is full of promises that confirm His love for you and His desire to give you His abundant life. His desire includes more than physical health for you; He wants to make you whole in your mind and spirit as well as through a personal relationship with His Son, Jesus Christ.

If you haven't met my best friend, Jesus, I would like to take this opportunity to introduce Him to you. It is very simple. If you are ready to let Him come into your life and become your best friend, all you need to do is sincerely pray this prayer:

> *Lord Jesus, I want to know You as my Savior and Lord. I believe You are the Son of God and that You died for my sins. I also believe You were raised from the dead and now sit at the right hand of the Father praying for me. I ask You to forgive me for my sins and change my heart so that I can be Your child and live with You eternally. Thank You for Your peace. Help me to walk with You so that I can begin to know You as my best friend and my Lord. Amen.*

If you have prayed this prayer, you have just made the most important decision of your life. I rejoice with you in your decision and your new relationship with Jesus. Please contact my publisher at pray4me@charismamedia.com so that we can send you some materials that will help you become established in your relationship with the Lord. We look forward to hearing from you.

NOTES

CHAPTER 2

1. "Water: How Much Should You Drink Every Day?," Mayo Clinic, October 12, 2022, https://www.mayoclinic.org/healthy-lifestyle/ nutrition-and-healthy-eating/in-depth/water/art-20044256.

2. Dana E. King, Arch G. Mainous III, and Carol A. Lambourne, "Trends in Dietary Fiber Intake in the United States, 1999–2008," *Journal of the Academy of Nutrition and Dietetics* 112, no. 5 (May 2012): 642–48, https://pubmed.ncbi.nlm.nih.gov/22709768/.

3. Diane Quagliani and Patricia Felt-Gunderson, "Closing America's Fiber Intake Gap," *American Journal of Lifestyle Medicine* 11, no. 1 (January– February 2017): 80–85, https://www.ncbi.nlm.nih.gov/pmc/articles/ PMC6124841/.

4. American Osteopathic Association, "Low Magnesium Levels Make Vitamin D Ineffective," ScienceDaily, February 26, 2018, https://www. sciencedaily.com/releases/2018/02/180226122548.htm.

5. U.S. Department of Agriculture and U.S. Department of Health and Human Services, "Appendix 1: Nutritional Goals for Age-Sex Groups," *2020–2025 Dietary Guidelines for Americans*, 9th ed., December 2020, 133, https://www.dietaryguidelines.gov/sites/default/files/2021-03/ Dietary_Guidelines_for_Americans-2020-2025.pdf.

6. M. A. Puertollano et al., "[Olive Oil, Immune System and Infection]," *Nutricion Hospitalaria* 25, no. 1 (January–February 2010): 1–8, https:// pubmed.ncbi.nlm.nih.gov/20204249/.

7. Gundry MD Team, "Dr. Gundry Diet Food List: A Comprehensive Lectin Free Diet Plan," Gundry MD, April 8, 2023, https://gundrymd. com/dr-gundry-diet-food-list/.

CHAPTER 3

1. Quagliani and Felt-Gunderson, "Closing America's Fiber Intake Gap."

2. Brian Krans, "The Health Benefits of Psyllium," Healthline, April 22, 2019, https://www.healthline.com/health/psyllium-health-benefits; Alisa Hrustic, "5 Signs You're Not Eating Enough Fiber," *Men's Health*, October 30, 2017, https://www.menshealth.com/nutrition/a19540392/ signs-of-low-fiber-diet/.

3. Maitreyi Raman, Angela Sirounis, and Jennifer Shrubsole, *The Complete Prebiotic and Probiotic Health Guide: A Vegetarian Plan for*

Balancing Your Gut Flora (Toronto: Robert Rose, 2015), 63–64; Krans, "The Health Benefits of Psyllium."

4. Cerner Multum, "*Lactobacillus acidophilus*," Drugs.com, June 1, 2020, https://www.drugs.com/mtm/lactobacillus-acidophilus.html.

5. Svetlana Sokovic Bajic et al., "GABA-Producing Natural Dairy Isolate From Artisanal Zlatar Cheese Attenuates Gut Inflammation and Strengthens Gut Epithelial Barrier *in Vitro*," *Frontiers in Microbiology* 10 (March 18, 2019): 527, https://www.ncbi.nlm.nih.gov/pmc/articles/PMC6431637/.

6. Erika Isolauri, "Probiotics for Infectious Diarrhoea," *Gut* 52, no. 3 (2003): 436–37, https://www.ncbi.nlm.nih.gov/pmc/articles/PMC1773578/.

7. Ryuzo Deguchi et al., "Effect of Pretreatment with *Lactobacillus gasseri* OLL2716 on First-Line *Helicobacter pylori* Eradication Therapy" *Journal of Gastroenterology and Hepatology* 27, no. 5 (November 18, 2011): 888–92, https://doi.org/10.1111/j.1440-1746.2011.06985.x.

8. Marlene Wullt et al., "*Lactobacillus plantarum* 299v Enhances the Concentrations of Fecal Short-Chain Fatty Acids in Patients with Recurrent *Clostridium difficile*–Associated Diarrhea," *Digestive Diseases and Sciences* 52, no. 9 (2007): 2082–86, https://pubmed.ncbi.nlm.nih.gov/17420953/; Cathy Wong, "The Benefits and Uses of *Lactobacillus plantarum*," Verywell Health, June 13, 2020, https://www.verywellhealth.com/lactobacillus-plantarum-benefits-uses-side-effects-4152035.

9. Isolauri, "Probiotics for Infectious Diarrhoea."

10. Francesco Savino et al., "Antagonistic Effect of *Lactobacillus* Strains Against Gas-Producing Coliforms Isolated from Colicky Infants," *BMC Microbiology* 11 (June 30, 2011): 157, https://www.ncbi.nlm.nih.gov/pmc/articles/PMC3224137/.

11. Evan Jerkunica, "What Is Probiotic *S. thermophilus*?," Probiotics.org, accessed August 26, 2020, https://probiotics.org/s-thermophilus/.

12. Lorena Ruiz et al., "Bifidobacteria and Their Molecular Communication with the Immune System," *Frontiers in Microbiology* 8 (December 4, 2017): 2345, https://www.ncbi.nlm.nih.gov/pmc/articles/PMC5722804/.

13. Kelli Hansen, "How to Use the Probiotic *Bifidobacterium infantis*," Healthline, May 17, 2017, https://www.healthline.com/health/bifidobacterium-infantis.

14. Toshitaka Odamaki et al., "Effect of the Oral Intake of Yogurt Containing *Bifidobacterium longum* BB536 on the Cell Numbers of Enterotoxigenic *Bacteroides fragilis* in Microbiota," *Anaerobe*

18, no. 1 (2012): 14–18, https://pubmed.ncbi.nlm.nih.gov/22138361/; Katie Stone, "Major Health Benefits of *Bifidobacterium longum*," Balance One, October 18, 2017, https://balanceone.com/blogs/news/bifidobacteriumlongum.

15. Evan Jerkunica, "B. Lactics Probiotics Supplementation Benefits," Probiotics.org, accessed August 26, 2020, https://probiotics.org/bifidobacterium-lactis/.

16. Cerner Multum, "*Saccharomyces boulardii lyo*," Drugs.com, November 26, 2019, https://www.drugs.com/mtm/saccharomyces-boulardii-lyo.html.

17. Raphael Kellman, *The Microbiome Breakthrough: Harness the Power of Your Gut Bacteria to Boost Your Mood and Heal Your Body* (New York: Da Capo Press, 2018), 112.

18. Robynne Chutkan, *The Microbiome Solution: A Radical New Way to Heal Your Body from the Inside Out* (New York: Avery, 2015), 170.

19. Crystal Raypole, "Can Probiotics Help With Depression?," Healthline, March 21, 2019, https://www.healthline.com/health/probioticsdepression.

20. Raypole, "Can Probiotics Help With Depression?"

21. Reza Ranuh et al., "Effect of the *Probiotic Lactobacillus plantarum* IS-10506 on BDNF and 5HT Stimulation: Role of Intestinal Microbiota on the Gut-Brain Axis," *Iranian Journal of Microbiology* 11, no. 2 (2019): 145–50, https://www.ncbi.nlm.nih.gov/pmc/articles/PMC6635314/.

22. Mary Jane Brown, "8 Health Benefits of Probiotics," Healthline, August 23, 2016, https://www.healthline.com/nutrition/8-health-benefits-ofprobiotics.

23. C. Han et al., "The Role of Probiotics in Lipopolysaccharide-Induced Autophagy in Intestinal Epithelial Cells," *Cellular Physiology and Biochemistry* 38, no. 6 (June 2016), https://www.karger.com/Article/Fulltext/445597.

24. Steven R. Gundry, *The Plant Paradox: The Hidden Dangers in "Healthy" Foods That Cause Disease and Weight Gain* (New York: HarperCollins, 2017), 144.

25. Limor Goren et al., "(-)-Oleocanthal and (-)-Oleocanthal-Rich Olive Oils Induce Lysosomal Membrane Permeabilization in Cancer Cells," *Plos One* (August 14, 2019), https://doi.org/10.1371/journal.pone.0216024.

Chapter 5

1. "Dietary Guidelines for Americans," USDA, December 2020, https://www.dietaryguidelines.gov/sites/default/files/2021-03/Dietary_Guidelines_for_Americans-2020-2025.pdf.

2. Jeff S. Volek and Stephen D. Phinney, *The Art and Science of Low Carbohydrate Performance* (Lexington, KY: Beyond Obesity, 2012), 7.

Chapter 6

1. Jacqueline D. Wright and Chia-Yih Wang, "Trends in Intake of Energy and Macronutrients in Adults From 1999–2000 Through 2007–2008," NCHS Brief, no. 49, November 2010, https://www.cdc.gov/nchs/data/databriefs/db49.pdf.

2. Ramón Estruch et al., "Primary Prevention of Cardiovascular Disease With a Mediterranean Diet Supplemented With Extra-Virgin Olive Oil or Nuts," *New England Journal of Medicine* 378, no. 25 (June 21, 2018): e34, https://doi.org/10.1056/nejmoa1800389.

3. "Fats," American Diabetes Association, accessed September 13, 2021, https://www.diabetes.org/healthy-living/recipes-nutrition/eating-well/fats.

4. Mayo Clinic Staff, "Trans Fat Is Double Trouble for Your Heart Health"; Vandana Dhaka et al., "Trans Fats—Sources, Health Risks and Alternative Approach—a Review," *Journal of Food Science Technology* 48, no. 5 (October 2011): 534–541, https://dx.doi.org/10.1007%2Fs13197-010-0225-8.

5. E. Patterson et al., "Health Implications of High Dietary Omega-6 Polyunsaturated Fatty Acids," *Journal of Nutrition and Metabolism* 2012, no. 539426 (2012), https://doi.org/10.1155/2012/539426.

6. M. J. Reed et al., "Free Fatty Acids: A Possible Regulator of the Available Oestradiol Fractions in Plasma," *Journal of Steroid Biochemistry* 24, no. 2 (February 1986): 657–659, https://doi.org/10.1016/0022-4731(86)90143-2; Karma L. Pearce and Kelton Tremellen, "The Effect of Macronutrients on Reproductive Hormones in Overweight and Obese Men: A Pilot Study," *Nutrients* 11, no. 12 (2019): 3059, https://doi.org/10.3390/nu11123059; P. C. Calder, "Polyunsaturated Fatty Acids, Inflammation, and Immunity," *Lipids* 36, no. 9 (September 2001): 1007–1024, https://doi.org/10.1007/s11745-001-0812-7; Urszula Radzikowska et al., "The Influence of Dietary Fatty Acids on Immune Responses," *Nutrients* 11, no. 12 (December 2019): 2990, https://dx.doi.org/10.3390%2Fnu11122990; Anamaria Balić et al., "Omega-3 Versus Omega-6 Polyunsaturated Fatty Acids

in the Prevention and Treatment of Inflammatory Skin Diseases," *International Journal of Molecular Sciences* 21, no. 3 (February 2020): 741, https://dx.doi.org/10.3390%2Fijms21030741.

7. Maria Azrad, Chelsea Turgeon, and Wendy Demark-Wahnefried, "Current Evidence Linking Polyunsaturated Fatty Acids With Cancer Risk and Progression," *Frontiers in Oncology* 3 (2013): 224, https://dx.doi.org/10.3389%2Ffonc.2013.00224.

8. Foundation staff, "Healthiest Cooking Oil Comparison Chart With Smoke Points and Omega 3 Fatty Acid Ratios," Baseline of Health Foundation, April 17, 2019, https://www.jonbarron.org/diet-and-nutrition/healthiest-cooking-oil-chart-smokepoints.

9. Will Cole, *Ketotarian* (New York: Avery, 2018), 21, https://www.amazon.com/Ketotarian-Mostly-Plant-Based-Cravings-Inflammation/dp/0525537171.

10. Mark Hyman, *The Pegan Diet* (New York: Little, Brown Spark, 2021), 64.

11. H. D. Karsten et al., "Vitamins A, E and Fatty Acid Composition of the Eggs of Caged Hens and Pastured Hens," *Renewable Agriculture and Food Systems* 25, no. 1 (2010): 45–54, https://doi.org/10.1017/S1742170509990214.

12. Suzanne Ryan, *Simply Keto* (Las Vegas: Victory Belt, 2017), 53.

13. "Grass-Fed Beef: Is It Good for You?," WebMD, accessed September 14, 2021, https://www.webmd.com/diet/grass-fed-beef-good-for-you#1.

14. Don Colbert, MD, *Dr. Colbert's Keto Zone Diet* (Franklin, TN: Worthy Books, 2017), 123.

15. Ryan, *Simply Keto*, 53.

16. Martha Clare Morris et al., "Consumption of Fish and N-3 Fatty Acids and Risk of Incident Alzheimer Disease," *Archives of Neurology* 60, no. 7 (July 2003): 940–946, https://doi.org/10.1001/archneur.60.7.940.

17. Hyman, *The Pegan Diet*, 65–66.

18. Hyman, *The Pegan Diet*, 42.

19. Hyman, *The Pegan Diet*, 45.

20. Hyman, *The Pegan Diet*, 46.

21. Hyman, *The Pegan Diet*, 21.

22. Hyman, *The Pegan Diet*, 46.

23. Piet A. van den Brandt and Leo J. Schouten, "Relationship of Tree Nut, Peanut and Peanut Butter Intake With Total and Cause-Specific Mortality: A Cohort Study and Meta-Analysis," *International Journal of Epidemiology* 44, no. 3 (2015): 1038–1049, https://doi.org/10.1093/ije/dyv039; Joan Sabaté, Keiji Oda, and Emilio Ros, "Nut Consumption

and Blood Lipid Levels: A Pooled Analysis of 25 Intervention Trials," *Archives of Internal Medicine* 170, no. 9 (May 10, 2010): 821–827, https://doi.org/10.1001/archinternmed.2010.79; Luc Djoussé, Tamara Rudich, and J. Michael Gaziano, "Nut Consumption and Risk of Hypertension in US Male Physicians," *Clinical Nutrition* 28, no. 1 (February 2009): 10–14, https://dx.doi.org/10.1016%2Fj.clnu.2008.08.005.

Chapter 7

1. Josh Axe, *Keto Diet* (New York: Little, Brown Spark, 2019), 15.
2. Mark Hyman, *Eat Fat, Get Thin* (New York: Little, Brown and Company, 2016), 75; Glen D. Lawrence, "Dietary Fats and Health: Dietary Recommendations in the Context of Scientific Evidence," *Advances in Nutrition* 4, no. 3 (May 2013): 294–302, https://doi.org/10.3945/an.113.003657.
3. Tingting Shang et al., "Protective Effects of Various Ratios of DHA/EPA Supplementation on High-Fat Diet-Induced Liver Damage in Mice," *Lipids in Health and Disease* 16, no. 1 (March 29, 2017): 65, https://doi.org/10.1186/s12944-017-0461-2.
4. "Vitamin Supplements: Hype or Help for Healthy Eating," American Heart Association, accessed September 10, 2021, https://www.heart.org/en/healthy-living/healthy-eating/eat-smart/nutrition-basics/vitamin-supplements-hype-or-help-forhealthy-eating?uid=1923.
5. EFSA Panel on Dietetic Products, Nutrition and Allergies (NDA), "Scientific Opinion on the Tolerable Upper Intake Level of Eicosapentaenoic Acid (EPA), Docosahexaenoic Acid (DHA) and Docosapentaenoic Acid (DPA)," *EFSA Journal* 10, no. 7 (July 27, 2012): 2815, https://doi.org/10.2903/j.efsa.2012.2815.

Chapter 8

1. Michel de Lorgeril et al., "Mediterranean Dietary Pattern in a Randomized Trial," *Archives of Internal Medicine* 158, no. 11 (1998): 1181–1187, https://doi.org/10.1001/archinte.158.11.1181.
2. Theodora Psaltopoulou et al., "Olive Oil Intake Is Inversely Related to Cancer Prevalence: A Systematic Review and a Meta-Analysis of 13800 Patients and 23340 Controls in 19 Observational Studies," *Lipids in Health and Disease* 10, no. 127 (2011), https://doi.org/10.1186/1476-511X-10-127.
3. Estefanía Toledo et al., "Mediterranean Diet and Invasive Breast Cancer Risk Among Women at High Cardiovascular Risk in the PREDIMED

Trial," *JAMA Internal Medicine* 175, no. 11 (2015): 1752–1760, https://doi.org/10.1001/jamainternmed.2015.4838.

4. Steven Masley, *The Mediterranean Method* (New York: Harmony Books, 2019), 25.

5. Hyman, *Eat Fat, Get Thin*, 216.

6. Klaas Vandepoele and Yves Van de Peer, "Exploring the Plant Transcriptome Through Phylogenetic Profiling," *Plant Physiology* 137 (January 2005): 31–42, http://bioinformatics.psb.ugent.be/pdf/klpoepph.pdf.

CHAPTER 9

1. Maria Cohut, "Intermittent Fasting May Have 'Profound Health Benefits,'" Medical News Today, May 1, 2018, https://www.medicalnewstoday.com/articles/321690.php?iacp.

2. Radhika V. Seimon et al., "Do Intermittent Diets Provide Physiological Benefits Over Continuous Diets for Weight Loss? A Systematic Review of Clinical Trials," *Molecular and Cellular Endocrinology* 418, no. 2 (December 15, 2015): 153–172, https://www.sciencedirect.com/science/article/pii/S0303720715300800?via%3Dihub.

3. Chris Kresser, "Intermittent Fasting: The Science Behind the Trend," Chris Kresser, March 25, 2019, https://chriskresser.com/intermittent-fasting-the-science-behind-the-trend/.

4. Kelsey Gabel et al., "Effects of 8-Hour Time Restricted Feeding on Body Weight and Metabolic Disease Risk Factors in Obese Adults: A Pilot Study," *Nutrition and Healthy Aging* 4, no. 4 (June 15, 2018): 345–353, https://content.iospress.com/articles/nutrition-and-healthy-aging/nha170036.

5. Aaron Kandola, "What Are the Benefits of Intermittent Fasting?," Medical News Today, November 7, 2018, https://www.medicalnewstoday.com/articles/323605.php.

6. Joe Sugarman, "Are There Any Proven Benefits to Fasting?," *John Hopkins Health Review* 3, no. 1 (Spring/Summer 2016), https://www.johnshopkinshealthreview.com/issues/springsummer-2016/articles/are-there-any-proven-benefits-to-fasting.

7. David Perlmutter, "Benefits of Intermittent Fasting for Your Brain and Body," Dr. Perlmutter, November 15, 2018, https://www.drperlmutter.com/benefits-of-intermittent-fasting/.

8. Kresser, "Intermittent Fasting."

9. Robert Krikorian et al., "Dietary Ketosis Enhances Memory in Mild Cognitive Impairment," *Neurobiology of Aging* 33, no. 2 (2012): 425. e19–27, https://www.ncbi.nlm.nih.gov/pmc/articles/PMC3116949/.

10. Kresser, "Intermittent Fasting"; Mark P. Mattson et al., "Intermittent Metabolic Switching, Neuroplasticity and Brain Health," *Nature Reviews: Neuroscience* 19, no. 2 (2018): 63–80, https://www.ncbi.nlm.nih.gov/pmc/articles/PMC5913738/.

11. Kresser, "Intermittent Fasting."

12. Emma Young, "Fasting May Protect Against Disease: Some Say It May Even Be Good for the Brain," *Washington Post*, December 31, 2012, https://www.washingtonpost.com/national/health-science/fasting-may-protect-against-disease-some-sayit-may-even-be-good-for-the-brain/2012/12/24/6e521ee8-3588-11e2-bb9b-288a310849ee_story.html?noredirect=on.

13. Sugarman, "Are There Any Proven Benefits to Fasting?"

14. Bronwen Martin, Mark P. Mattson, and Stuart Maudsley, "Caloric Restriction and Intermittent Fasting: Two Potential Diets for Successful Brain Aging," *Ageing Research Reviews* 5, no. 3 (August 2006), 332–353, https://www.ncbi.nlm.nih.gov/pmc/articles/PMC2622429/.

15. "Risk Factors for Type 2 Diabetes," National Institute of Diabetes and Digestive and Kidney Diseases, November 2016, https://www.niddk.nih.gov/health-information/diabetes/overview/risk-factors-type-2-diabetes.

16. "Adult Obesity Facts," Centers for Disease Control and Prevention, accessed August 31, 2023, https://www.cdc.gov/obesity/data/adult.html; "Overweight and Obesity Statistics," National Institute of Diabetes and Digestive and Kidney Diseases, accessed August 31, 2023, https://www.niddk.nih.gov/health-information/health-statistics/overweight-obesity.

17. "The Cost of Diabetes," American Diabetes Association, accessed September 17, 2019, https://www.diabetes.org/resources/statistics/cost-diabetes.

18. Mark P. Mattson, Valter D. Longo, and Michelle Harvie, "Impact of Intermittent Fasting on Health and Disease Processes," *Ageing Research Reviews* 39 (2017): 46–58, https://www.ncbi.nlm.nih.gov/pmc/articles/PMC5411330/.

19. Kandola, "What Are the Benefits of Intermittent Fasting?"; Mattson, Longo, and Harvie, "Impact of Intermittent Fasting on Health and Disease Processes."

20. Elizabeth F. Sutton et al., "Early Time-Restricted Feeding Improves Insulin Sensitivity, Blood Pressure, and Oxidative Stress Even Without Weight Loss in Men With Prediabetes," *Cell Metabolism* 27, no. 6

(June 5, 2018): 1159–1160, https://www.sciencedirect.com/science/article/pii/S1550413118302535; Mattson, Longo, and Harvie, "Impact of Intermittent Fasting on Health and Disease Processes."

21. Kandola, "What Are the Benefits of Intermittent Fasting?"

22. Naomi Whittel, "The 12 Important Benefits of Autophagy," Naomi Whittel, accessed September 17, 2019, https://www.naomiwhittel.com/the-12-important-benefits-of-autophagy/.

23. Miroslava Cedikova et al., "Mitochondria in White, Brown, and Beige Adipocytes," *Stem Cells International* (2016): 6067349, https://www.ncbi.nlm.nih.gov/pmc/articles/PMC4814709/.

24. Whittel, "The 12 Important Benefits of Autophagy."

25. Daniele Lettieri-Barbato et al., "Time-Controlled Fasting Prevents Aging-Like Mitochondrial Changes Induced by Persistent Dietary Fat Overload in Skeletal Muscle," *PLoS One* 13, no. 5 (May 9, 2018): e0195912, https://www.ncbi.nlm.nih.gov/pmc/articles/PMC5942780/.

Chapter 10

1. Y. Handa et al., "Estrogen Concentrations in Beef and Human Hormone-Dependent Cancers," *Annals of Oncology* 20, no. 9 (September 1, 2009): 1610–1611, https://doi.org/10.1093/annonc/mdp381.

2. R. Jayaraj et al., "Organochlorine Pesticides, Their Toxic Effects on Living Organisms, and Their Fate in the Environment," *Interdisciplinary Toxicology* 2016, Vol. 9 (3–4): 90–100, https://sciendo.com/abstract/journals/intox/9/3-4/article-p90.xml.

3. Dale E. Bredesen, *The End of Alzheimer's* (New York: Avery, 2017), 131.

4. Erica Zelfand, "Pregnenolone for Memory, Mood, and Brain Health," Allergy Research Group, 2019, https://www.allergyresearchgroup.com/blog/pregnenolone-and-memory.

5. Thomas Guilliams, "Re-assessing the Notion of 'Pregnenolone Steal,'" ZRT Blog, June 21, 2017, https://www.zrtlab.com/blog/archive/reassessing-pregnenolone-steal.

6. "Breast Cancer in Young Women," Centers for Disease Control and Prevention, accessed September 20, 2022, https://www.cdc.gov/cancer/breast/young_women/bringyourbrave/breast_cancer_young_women/index.htm#:~:text=Breast%20cancer%20is%20the%20most,under%20the%20age%20of%2045.

7. Bredesen, *The End of Alzheimer's*, 51.

8. Anna-Karin Lennartsson et al., "Perceived Stress at Work Is Associated With Lower Levels of DHEA-S," *PLoS One* 8, no. 8 (2013): e72460, journals.plos.org/plosone/article?id=10.1371/journal.pone.0072460.

9. Gary Small and Gigi Vorgan, *The Memory Bible* (New York: Hachette Go, 2021), 175.

10. Avrum Bluming and Carol Tavris, *Estrogen Matters* (New York: Little, Brown Spark, 2018), 237.

11. Marianne Thvilum et al., "Increased Risk of Dementia in Hypothyroidism: A Danish Nationwide Register-Based Study," *Clinical Endocrinology* 94, no. 6 (June 2021): 1017–1024, https://doi.org/10.1111/cen.14424.

CHAPTER 11

1. Mark Starr, MD, *Hypothyroidism Type 2* (Columbia, MO: Mark Starr Trust, 2005), 1.

2. Broda O. Barnes, *Hypothyroidism: The Unsuspected Illness* (New York: Harper & Row, 1939).

3. Gary Donovitz, *Age Healthier, Live Happier* (Winter Park, FL: Celebrity Press, 2015), 57.

4. Janie A. Bowthorpe, *Stop the Thyroid Madness* (Castle Rock, CO: Laughing Grape Publishing, 2008), 50.

5. Starr, *Hypothyroidism Type 2*, 70.

6. Janie A. Bowthorpe, *Stop the Thyroid Madness II* (Castle Rock, CO: Laughing Grape Publishing, 2014), 83.

7. "Iodine Deficiency," American Thyroid Association, accessed September 27, 2018, https://www.thyroid.org/iodine-deficiency/.

8. Karla Robinson, MD, "Why Synthroid Is Among the Most Prescribed Medications in the US," GoodRx Health, October 18, 2022, https://www.goodrx.com/blog/why-synthroid-is-the-most-prescribed-drug-in-the-us/.

9. Yusuf "JP" Saleeby, in Bowthorpe, *Stop the Thyroid Madness II*, 65.

10. Saleeby in Bowthorpe, *Stop the Thyroid Madness II*.

11. Bowthorpe, *Stop the Thyroid Madness II*, 246.

CHAPTER 12

1. A. R. Genazzani et al., "Long-Term Low-Dose Dehydroepiandrosterone Replacement Therapy in Aging Males With Partial Androgen Deficiency," *Aging Male* 7, no. 2 (June 2004): 133–43, https://www.ncbi.nlm.nih.gov/pubmed/15672938.

2. Paul J. Rosch, "America's Leading Adult Health Problem," *USA Magazine*, May 1991.

Chapter 13

1. Will Brink, "Preventing Sarcopenia," *Life Extension*, January 2007, http://www.lifeextension.com/Magazine/2007/1/report_muscle/Page-01?p=1.
2. Kathy C. Maupin, *The Secret Female Hormone* (Carlsbad, CA: Hay House, 2014), xxi.
3. Donovitz, *Age Healthier, Live Happier*, 75.
4. "Progesterone," Laboratory Corporation of America Holdings, accessed September 7, 2023, https://www.labcorp.com/tests/004317/progesterone.
5. K. M. Webber, "The Contribution of Luteinizing Hormone to Alzheimer Disease Pathogenesis," *Clinical Medicine and Research* 5, no. 3 (October 2007): 177–83, https://doi.org/10.3121/cmr.2007.741.
6. Maupin, *The Secret Female Hormone*, 125.

Chapter 14

1. Jay Campbell, *The Definitive Testosterone Replacement Therapy Manual* (n.p.: Archangel Ink, 2015), 39.
2. "Educational Commentary—Testosterone and Sex-Hormone Binding Globulin," American Proficiency Institute, accessed September 27, 2018, http://www.apipt.com/Reference/Commentary/2013Achem.pdf.
3. C. Ohlsson et al., "High Serum Testosterone Is Associated With Reduced Risk of Cardiovascular Events in Elderly Men. The MrOS (Osteoporotic Fractures in Men) Study in Sweden," *Journal of the American College of Cardiology* 58, no. 16 (October 11, 2011): 1674–81, https://doi.org/10.1016/j.jacc.2011.07.019.
4. Juan Augustine Galindo Jr., "Normal Estradiol Levels in Men," Testosterone Centers of Texas, September 27, 2016, https://tctmed.com/normal-estradiol-levels/.
5. "Educational Commentary—Testosterone and Sex-Hormone Binding Globulin," American Proficiency Institute, accessed September 27, 2018, http://www.api-pt.com/Reference/Commentary/2013Achem.pdf.
6. K. M. Lakshman et al., "The Effects of Injected Testosterone Dose and Age on the Conversion of Testosterone to Estradiol and Dihydrotestosterone in Young and Older Men," *Journal of Clinical Endocrinology and Metabolism* 95, no. 8 (August 2010): 3955–64, https://doi.org/10.1210/jc.2010-0102.
7. "A Population-Level Decline in Serum Testosterone Levels in American Men," *Journal of Clinical Endocrinology and Metabolism* 92, no. 1 (January 2007): 196–202, https://doi.org/10.1210/jc.2006-1375.

8. P. G. Cohen, "Aromatase, Adiposity, Aging and Disease. The Hypogonadal-Metabolic-Atherogenic-Disease and Aging Connection," *Medical Hypotheses* 56, no. 6 (June 2001): 702–8, https://doi.org/10.1054/mehy.2000.1169; P. G. Cohen, "The Hypogonadal-Obesity Cycle: Role of Aromatase in Modulating the Testosterone-Estradiol Shunt—a Major Factor in the Genesis of Morbid Obesity," *Medical Hypotheses* 52, no. 1 (January 1999): 49–51, https://doi.org/10.1054/mehy.1997.0624.

Chapter 15

1. Sanjay Gupta, *Keep Sharp* (New York: Simon & Shuster, 2021), 59.
2. Gupta, *Keep Sharp*, 61.
3. Dale E. Bredesen, MD, *The End of Alzheimer's Program* (New York: Avery, 2020), 97–98.
4. Bredesen, *The End of Alzheimer's*, 42.
5. Bredesen, *The End of Alzheimer's*, 31.
6. Small and Vorgan, *The Memory Bible*, 14.

Chapter 16

1. Oliver E. Owen and Richard W. Hanson, "Ketone Bodies," Science Direct, accessed September 13, 2021, https://www.sciencedirect.com/topics/neuroscience/ketone-bodies.
2. Matthew K. Taylor et al., "Feasibility and Efficacy Data From a Ketogenic Diet Intervention in Alzheimer's Disease," *Alzheimer's & Dementia* (NY) 4 (2018): 28–36, https://doi.org/10.1016%2Fj.trci.2017.11.002.
3. T. B. Vanitallie et al., "Treatment of Parkinson Disease With Diet-Induced Hyperketonemia: A Feasibility Study," *Neurology* 64, no. 4 (February 22, 2005): 728–730, https://doi.org/10.1212/01.wnl.0000152046.11390.45.
4. Bredesen, *The End of Alzheimer's Program*, 74.
5. Bredesen, *The End of Alzheimer's Program*, 114.
6. Bredesen, *The End of Alzheimer's Program*, 122.
7. Bredesen, *The End of Alzheimer's Program*, 302–303.
8. Gupta, *Keep Sharp*, 88.
9. Bredesen, *The End of Alzheimer's Program*, 154–155.
10. Freydis Hjalmarsdottir, "How Much Omega-3 Should You Take Per Day?," Healthline, December 15, 2019, https://www.healthline.com/nutrition/how-much-omega-3.

11.   Yuusuke Saitsu et al., "Improvement of Cognitive Functions by Oral Intake of Hericium Erinaceus," *Biomedical Research* 40, no. 4 (2019): 125–131, https://doi.org/10.2220/biomedres.40.125.

12.   Bredesen, *The End of Alzheimer's Program*, 135.

13.   Small and Vorgan, *The Memory Bible*, 149.

14.   Susan J. Hewlings and Douglas S. Kalman, "Curcumin: A Review of Its Effects on Human Health," *Foods* 6, no. 10 (2017): 92, https://doi.org/10.3390/foods6100092.

15.   Gary W. Small et al., "Memory and Brain Amyloid and Tau Effects of a Bioavailable Form of Curcumin in Non-Demented Adults: A Double-Blind, Placebo-Controlled 18-Month Trial," *American Journal of Geriatric Psychiatry* 26, no. 3 (March 1, 2018): P266–P277, https://doi.org/10.1016/j.jagp.2017.10.010.

16.   Bredesen, *The End of Alzheimer's Program*, 183.

17.   Bredesen, *The End of Alzheimer's*, 103.

18.   Bredesen, *The End of Alzheimer's*, 199–121.

19.   Traci Stein, "A Genetic Mutation That Can Affect Mental & Physical Health," *Psychology Today*, September 5, 2014, https://www.psychologytoday.com/us/blog/the-integrationist/201409/geneticmutation-can-affect-mental-physical-health.

20.   Jim Kwik, *Limitless* (Carlsbad, CA: Hay House, 2020), 38.

21.   Joseph Pizzorno, *The Toxin Solution* (New York: HarperOne, 2017), 112–114, 119–120, 126.

22.   Bredesen, *The End of Alzheimer's Program*, 156.

23.   Small and Vorgan, *The Memory Bible*, 143.

24.   Small and Vorgan, *The Memory Bible*, 154–155.

25.   Bredesen, *The End of Alzheimer's Program*, 12.

26.   Bredesen, *The End of Alzheimer's Program*, 200.

27.   Alessandra Berry et al., "NGF, Brain and Behavioral Plasticity," *Neural Plasticity* (2012): 784040, https://doi.org/10.1155%2F2012%2F784040.

28.   Small and Vorgan, *The Memory Bible*, 153.

29.   Anthony G. Pacholko and Lane K. Bekar, "Lithium Orotate: A Superior Option for Lithium Therapy?," *Brain and Behavior* 11, no. 8 (August 2021): e2262, https://doi.org/10.1002%2Fbrb3.2262.

30.   Lars Vedel Kessing et al., "Association of Lithium in Drinking Water With the Incidence of Dementia," *JAMA Psychiatry* 74, no. 10 (2017): 1005–1010, https://doi.org/10.1001/jamapsychiatry.2017.2362.

31.   Young-Sung Kim et al., "Neuroprotective Effects of Magnesium L-Threonate in a Hypoxic Zebrafish Model," *BMC Neuroscience* 21,

no. 1 (June 26, 2020): 29, https://doi.org/10.1186/s12868-020-00580-6; Aparna Ann Mathew and Rajitha Panonnummal, "'Magnesium'—the Master Cation—as a Drug—Possibilities and Evidences," *Biometals* 34, no. 5 (2021): 955–986, https://doi.org/10.1007%2Fs10534-021-00328-7.

CHAPTER 17

1. Shalini Paruthi et al., "Recommended Amount of Sleep for Pediatric Populations: A Consensus Statement of the American Academy of Sleep Medicine," *Journal of Clinical Sleep Medicine* 12, no. 6 (June 15, 2016): 785–786, https://doi.org/10.5664%2Fjcsm.5866; Anne G. Wheaton et al., "Sleep Duration and Injury-Related Risk Behaviors Among High School Students—United States, 2007–2013," *Morbidity and Mortality Weekly Report* 65, no. 13 (April 8, 2016): 337–341, http://dx.doi.org/10.15585/mmwr.mm6513a1.

2. Jeffrey M. Jones, "In U.S., 40% Get Less Than Recommended Amount of Sleep," Gallup, December 19, 2013, https://news.gallup.com/poll/166553/less-recommended-amount-sleep.aspx.

3. Bredesen, *The End of Alzheimer's Program*, 45.

4. Gupta, *Keep Sharp*, 137.

5. Bredesen, *The End of Alzheimer's Program*, 214.

6. Gupta, *Keep Sharp*, 140–141.

7. Bredesen, *The End of Alzheimer's Program*, 214.

8. "Sleep and Sleep Disorder Statistics," American Sleep Association, accessed August 14, 2022, https://www.sleepassociation.org/aboutsleep/sleep-statistics/.

9. Bredesen, *The End of Alzheimer's Program*, 217.

10. Bredesen, *The End of Alzheimer's Program*, 222.

11. Robert M. Sapolsky, *Why Zebras Don't Get Ulcers*, 3rd edition (New York: Henry Holt & Company, 2004), 210.

12. Sapolsky, *Why Zebras Don't Get Ulcers*, 213.

13. Bredesen, *The End of Alzheimer's Program*, 228.

14. Small and Vorgan, *The Memory Bible*, 58.

15. Gupta, *Keep Sharp*, 108.

16. Gupta, *Keep Sharp*, 108.

17. Small and Vorgan, *The Memory Bible*, 60–61.

18. Gupta, *Keep Sharp*, 101.

19. Bredesen, *The End of Alzheimer's Program*, 200.

20. "Table 25. Participation in Leisure-Time Aerobic and Muscle-Strengthening Activities That Meet the Federal 2008 Physical Activity Guidelines for Americans Among Adults Aged 18 and Over, by Selected Characteristics: United States, Selected Years 1998–2018," Centers for Disease Control and Prevention, 2019, https://www.cdc.gov/nchs/data/hus/2019/025-508.pdf.

21. Small and Vorgan, *The Memory Bible*, 173.

22. Peter Elwood et al., "Healthy Lifestyles Reduce the Incidence of Chronic Diseases and Dementia: Evidence From the Caerphilly Cohort Study," *PLoS One* 8, no. 12 (December 9, 2013): e81877, https://doi.org/10.1371/journal.pone.0081877.

23. Bredesen, *The End of Alzheimer's Program*, 203.

24. David C. Peritz et al., "The Role of Stress Testing in the Older Athlete," American College of Cardiology, November 6, 2017, https://www.acc.org/latest-in-cardiology/articles/2017/11/06/10/32/the-role-of-stresstesting-in-the-older-athlete#.

25. "Coronary Artery Disease—Coronary Heart Disease," American Heart Association, accessed October 20, 2022, https://www.heart.org/en/health-topics/consumer-healthcare/what-is-cardiovascular-disease/coronary-artery-disease.

26. Phillip Nieto, "Cognitive Decline Can Be Avoided With Simple Everyday Exercises, New Study Suggests," Fox News, August 3, 2022, https://www.foxnews.com/health/cognitive-decline-avoided-simpleeverday-exercises-new-study-suggests.

27. Pedro F. Saint-Maurice et al., "Association of Leisure-Time Physical Activity Across the Adult Life Course With All-Cause and Cause-Specific Mortality," *JAMA Network Open* 2, no. 3 (March 1, 2019): e190355, https://doi.org/10.1001/jamanetworkopen.2019.0355.

28. Brian Downer et al., "The Relationship Between Midlife and Late Life Alcohol Consumption, APOE e4 and the Decline in Learning and Memory Among Older Adults," *Alcohol and Alcoholism* 49, no. 1 (January 2014): 17–22, https://doi.org/10.1093%2Falcalc%2Fagt144.

Appendix B

1. "ALCAT," Perkins Chiropractic Clinic, accessed September 17, 2019, https://www.perkinschiropractic.net/wp-content/uploads/2017/04/ALCAT_INFO.

INDEX

THANK YOU FOR READING
DR. COLBERT'S HEALTH ZONE ESSENTIALS

I hope this book has provided you with applicable insight and solutions to restore your body from the ailments plaguing you. I pray you have been equipped with the steps needed to add vitality to your life for years to come. If you haven't read the complete Zone series, be sure to check out my other books to learn more about how you can live a life of wellness.

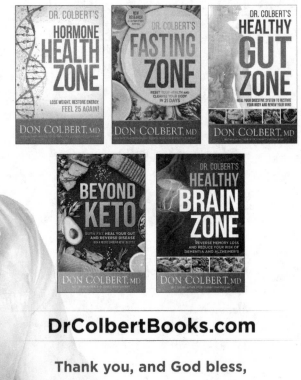

DrColbertBooks.com

Thank you, and God bless,

Thank you, and God bless,

SILOAM